Diet in Sport

Wilf Paish

Second edition published 1989 by
A & C Black (Publishers) Ltd
35 Bedford Row, London WC1R 4JH

First edition published 1979 by
EP Publishing Limited, West Yorkshire

ISBN 0 7136 5739 1

A CIP catalogue record for this book is
available from the British Library

Printed and bound in Great Britain by
Courier International

Contents

About the author

Wilf Paish trained as a teacher of physical education at Borough Road College and Carnegie College of Physical Education, Leeds. After teaching for a number of years he took up an appointment as a National Athletics Coach in 1964, and has been involved in that occupation ever since.

He has travelled widely to all major athletics fixtures and has been a team coach at the Olympic Games, Commonwealth Games and European Championships. In this capacity he has mixed with sportspeople, trainers, coaches and sports scientists from all over the world.

His interest in diet in sport started when he tried to study the ways of reducing the advantages which foreign athletes appeared to have over British athletes when involved in international competition. The study led to a deeper understanding of sports science, of which nutrition is just one aspect. He has lectured on the subject at international symposia and has written extensively on this as well as most other aspects of sports science.

Wilf Paish is essentially a practical man, totally involved in the day-to-day training of top athletes, including world record holders and an Olympic champion. He has successfully helped in the guidance of Halifax Rugby league football club to a division one championship and success at the Wembley Cup final. He is also a consultant to a number of leading soccer clubs.

Wilf's interest in education is widely recognised. He directs many in-service courses for teachers, and was involved as a consultant in the setting up of G.C.S.E. physical education. He visits schools to lecture on specific aspects of this syllabus and on health-related fitness.

Introduction

Sport is merely a challenge, a vehicle for exploring one's inner desires and ambitions. Just as the mountain is there to be climbed, so too are the other barriers in sport there to be conquered. Some people take part in sport as a healthy leisure activity; others wish to aspire to greater heights and join the ranks of the elite. However, once the challenge has been accepted, most wish to achieve their maximum potential by participating at the highest possible level, commensurate with their endowed ability or commitment. In their pursuit of excellence sportsmen and women subject their bodies to extreme levels of stress, undergo very strenuous training to achieve peak levels of fitness, seek the advice of coaches to improve performance techniques and take advantage of all that sports science can offer. Once a performer reaches this level of commitment, he or she recognises that no stone can remain unturned – it just might reveal the magic formula that could help tip the balance against rivals.

In truth, there is no magic formula. Success in sport is directly related to the amount of work, thought and preparation that one is prepared to invest. Very high levels of performance, many of them inflicted by the Eastern bloc nations, make it essential that we 'join them' at least in following their very thorough approach in preparing for their sport.

In searching for the magic formula, most sportsmen and women seldom look farther than a modification of their training programme, style of play, etc., often to bring them in line with a vogue, or a current champion. Very few are more basic and look at the simple raw materials for producing the energy they are continually expending. An analogy with the motor-car might help to give the reader a clearer understanding of the situation. There is little point in tuning the engine of a high-performance sports car only to put two-star petrol in the tank. Instead, high-octane fuels are used to give the best results and to reward the labours involved. The human engine can be finely tuned by careful training and preparation; to give of its best it, too, requires high-octane fuel which can only be obtained from the food eaten.

One still hears of outstanding sportsmen and women following the Victorian ideas of such concoctions as raw eggs and sherry or massive beefsteaks as pre-event meals. Nutrition for sport is full of such fads and fallacies. The enthusiast must be on guard against the

5

'quacks' in this field who recommend a particular beverage or food for commercial gains. There is a very strong case for the dietician, the trainer, the coach and the performer to pool their ideas. Only then can the true problem be investigated.

Frequently, dieticians and doctors suggest that the normal diet is adequate for the average person. However, it is difficult to establish what   a normal diet is and certainly the top class sportsperson cannot be classed as average. Indeed, the elite performer is a very unique person who comes from a group representing less than .00003% of the population.

It is hoped that this text will stimulate the reader into further study by providing the necessary background information. In some cases it can provide all of the information necessary to understand and apply this particular science and so, we hope, enhance levels of performance in sport.

The final section of the book gives an outline of the modern methods involved in training for sport. In so doing, it could provide the workshop manual for tuning and refuelling the human engine, so aiding to the greatest possible extent those who wish to achieve excellence in their chosen sport.

1
Digestion – food categories, vitamins and minerals

In order to function as living organisms the cells of the body are continually using energy. Even when the body is completely at rest, for example, during deep sleep, the essential functions of life must continue. Energy is a property of matter that cannot be created or destroyed. It is merely converted from one form to another with the sun being the original source. This basic form of energy is passed on to us, in order to maintain life, from the food which we eat. However, before the meat, vegetables, dairy products, etc. which we consume during meals can be utilised as a form of energy, they must undergo a complicated series of changes to be converted to a material which the cells of the body can use. Again, the analogy of the human body and the motor-car engine may aid the understanding of the process. Crude oil, direct from the well, would not burn in the engine. Instead, it must go through a refining process long before it is put into the petrol tank of the car. In this respect, the human machine has a significant advantage over the man-made comparison – it has its own built-in refinery.

The refining process is initiated as soon as the food is placed in the mouth. The action of mastication, combined with certain chemicals contained in our saliva, starts off a series of reactions which is continued along the length of the digestive tract until the food is converted into a substance which can be absorbed directly into the bloodstream and transported to the active cells to provide its energy for life.

While it is not the intention of this book to delve too deeply into the process of digestion, a simple understanding is essential for the reader to appreciate the finer aspects of sports nutrition.

The process by which food is taken into the body, digested and absorbed is known as alimentation and it takes place in the alimentary canal. The canal is about 26 feet (8 metres) long and consists of the mouth, throat, oesophagus, stomach, small intestine

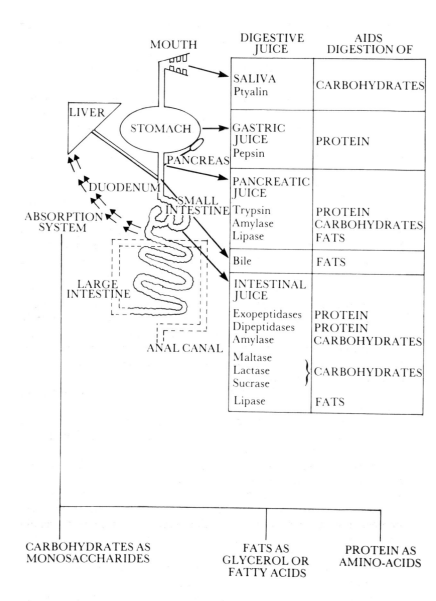

Diagram 1 shows the digestive process schematically

and large intestine. The alimentary canal is mainly composed of a four-layer tissue, one of the layers being smooth muscle which produces the movement of the food along the canal. As well as the simple digestive glands, which are contained in the walls of the canal, there are many other glands which pour their secretions along ducts into the alimentary canal. The digestive juices, as they are known, are composed mainly of water, in which the enzymes responsible for digestion are dissolved.

Digestion commences in the mouth where mastication takes place – the food is mixed with a lubricant, saliva. Saliva also contains an enzyme, ptyalin, which starts to break down starches into simpler starches. Once the food has been ground up and mixed with saliva, it is formed into a compact mass known as a bolus. The bolus takes up a position in the back of the throat and a reflex action draws the food mass into the oesophagus. A peristaltic action, set up by alternate contraction and relaxation of the muscular linings, propels the bolus towards the stomach. It takes on average about five seconds for the food to pass to the stomach, though dry foods take longer and the passage of liquids is almost instantaneous.

When the food enters the stomach, pepsin, which digests protein, is secreted and the nervous system is stimulated to produce gastric juice via glands situated in the linings of the stomach. The peristaltic action churns the food in the stomach, mixing it with the digestive enzymes. Food stays in the stomach for between two and four hours after a meal; it is then ejected into the small intestine, through the pyloric sphincter. At this stage the food forms an acid chyme.

Only water, alcohol and certain drugs are absorbed into the bloodstream from the stomach.

Once the acid chyme enters the small intestine it is neutralised by three alkaline digestive juices: pancreatic juice, bile and intestinal juice.

Pancreatic juice is the secretion of the pancreas. It contains several digestive enzymes, the most commonly known being trypsin, lipase and amylase. Trypsin aids in the digestion of proteins, lipase breaks down fats to fatty acids and glycerol and amylase break down starches into simpler compounds. The pancreas also secretes insulin directly into the blood. In the main, the action of the pancreas is controlled by hormones.

Bile is the secretion of special cells in the liver. It does not contain any digestive enzymes but aids in the digestion of fats.

Intestinal juice contains enzymes which are produced by a tissue breakdown of the cells lining the small intestine. The enzymes produced break down protein into amino-acids. Maltase, lactase and sucrase complete the breakdown of starches etc. into monosaccharides, while lipase completes the digestion of fats.

Most of the products of digestion are absorbed through the wall of the small intestine into the blood, by diffusion. By the time the chyme leaves the small intestine most of the nutrients have been absorbed. Carbohydrates are absorbed directly as monosaccharides, glucose and galactose. Fructose is absorbed by diffusion when there is a difference in its concentration between the intestine and the blood. Protein is absorbed direct as amino-acids, and fats as glycerol and fatty acids. Bile plays an intricate part in the absorption of in-completely digested fats.

The absorption of mineral salts, water and iron, when it is re-quired, takes place direct from the small intestine.

Only water and certain mineral salts are absorbed in the large intestine. Gradually along the length of the large intestine the water from the chyme is absorbed, leaving the hard faeces which are excreted during defecation.

Even this very brief study of the digestive system has necessitated the use of the terms carbohydrates, fats and proteins since these are the three basic chemical groups into which food can conveniently be categorised. In simpler terms, they are all compounds of carbon, hydrogen and oxygen and, in the case of protein, nitrogen.

Carbohydrates

As the word suggests, carbohydrates are compounds of carbon, hydrogen and oxygen, the ratio of the last two being two to one, as in water. Carbohydrates can exist in the form of simple sugars, such as glucose or fructose, or as compounds of these simple sugars to form complex molecules of starches. The body relies upon carbohydrates for its quick supply of energy. While both fats and proteins can also be used for energy, the body prefers the use of carbohydrates, especially during exercise, because of their more efficient metabolism. They are an instant source of energy as they can be stored in both muscle and the liver in the form of glycogen. However, it must be emphasised that this store is very small, in the region of about 2,500 Calories – enough to satisfy the energy requirements of a fairly sedentary person for one day. It must also be emphasised that carbohydrates are not an essential source of energy – they are just the quickest and cheapest. It is theoretically possible for the body to function without a supply of carbohydrates, as they do not provide any essential intermediary compounds, nor do they bind vitamins. So one can say that for sport they are just convenient.

Fats

Fats, like carbohydrates, contain carbon, hydrogen and oxygen. However, the hydrogen to oxygen ratio is not two to one because this factor varies according to the degree of 'saturation'. Compared with carbohydrates, fats have a relatively low oxygen content: hence they have a high energy potential, producing about two and a half times as many Calories on a weight basis. However, as far as sport is concerned they are inefficient because of their greater oxygen usage in the metabolic process. Even so, fats form the greatest store of energy within the body. For example, the body of an average young man is composed of about 16 per cent fat, which has a potential energy yield of 100,000 Calories, sufficient to last a sedentary person for several months.

The fats which we eat can be derived from both animal and vegetable sources. Those of plant origin are 'unsaturated', while the 'saturated' variety come from an animal source. The body requires a minimum amount of fatty acids to enable the kidneys and skin to function correctly and to transport the fat soluble vitamins (A, D, E and K) and they have an intricate function in the homeostatic effect of hormones. If one adds to this the thermo-insulatory effect of fat, its mechanical protection and its cosmetic function, its importance in life will soon be realised. However, it is generally estimated that man consumes at least 50 per cent more fat than is required, and this can have a detrimental effect upon health, particularly when a diet is excessive in fats of animal derivation. The main problem is that man has developed an appetite for animal fats, probably associated with the euphoric effect caused by their slow transit through the digestive system.

Proteins

Proteins are compounds which contain nitrogen in addition to the carbon, hydrogen and oxygen common to the other two categories, together with certain essential minerals. They are the body's only source of nitrogen and hence they are a prerequisite of life. The cells of the body are composed mainly of protein, which is constantly undergoing changes, and hence it is constantly needed to build new tissue and repair old tissue.

Proteins are composed of amino-acids (small molecules containing nitrogen). There are about twenty-eight known amino-acids, of which the body only requires eight. These are known as essential amino-acids and must be contained in the diet. The body is capable of synthesising the non-essential amino-acids, so they are of secondary importance.

The source for carbohydrates and fats is fairly obvious but the dietary presence of protein is frequently debated and many people develop an obsession for foods which they believe to contain the vital compound. In 1956, the United Nations Committee for food and agriculture rated the most common sources of protein in rank order. Eggs were found to contain the best balance of 'essential' amino-acids, and were given a 100 per cent rating. The other foods were rated in comparison to eggs, as follows:

eggs	100%
fish/meat	70%
soya beans	69%
milk	60%
rice	56%
corn	41%

Equally confusing is the amount of protein that should be taken daily. Even fairly reliable sources seem to contradict each other and values ranging from 25 grams to 125 grams per day are recommended by the various groups of research workers. Misunderstanding could arise from the fact that dietary requirements are proportional to lean body mass and as such should be given in grams per kilogram of bodyweight. Research work from an Eastern European source suggests values 0.5 g/kg, which indicates that a person weighing 60 kg or 134 lb needs in the region of 30 grams of protein per day. This tends to favour the lower limit of the range given previously and is supported by the recommendation of the League of Nations Committee in 1936, which was that the body required 1 gram of protein for every kilogram of adult bodyweight and 4 g/kg for a child.

The only essential feature is that the delicate nitrogen balance of the body must be kept, and the dietary intakes must allow for this.

Vitamins

Although the study of vitamins has been in progress now for about a century, few people know precisely what they are, or what they do. A fairly safe and simple idea is to regard them as the catalyst of nutritional chemistry. They speed up, or make more efficient, the digestive process which converts our foods to substances which can be used directly in the metabolic process.

Basically, vitamins are divided into two groups: fat-soluble – those which occur and dissolve in fat, namely vitamins A, D, E and K; and water-soluble – those which dissolve in water, namely vitamin B and C groups.

Vitamin A

Vitamin A can be taken directly into the body through one of the fish liver oils or indirectly via the carotene in vegetables and fruit. This substance is converted to vitamin A in the intestine, and is stored in the liver. For the conversion process to take place vitamin E must be present, so illustrating the dependence of vitamins upon each other.

It is suggested that vitamin A is essential for the well-being of all epithelial tissue. This tissue is found in most parts of the body including the skin and the respiratory, endocrine and nervous systems and its presence is thus essential for healthy life.

However, unless the diet is very low in fats it is most unlikely that the body will be deficient in this vitamin. It must also be stressed that large doses of vitamin A are toxic.

Vitamin B

This is a 'complex' of vitamins all related to one another in certain ways. As they are water-soluble they cannot be stored in the body, hence the need for a daily intake.

Thiamin (Vitamin B_1)

This is present in wheat-germ, which unfortunately is destroyed in the refining process of most flours. Vitamin B_1 plays an essential role in carbohydrate metabolism, acting as a coenzyme for the oxidisation of pyruvic acid (see p. 26).

Riboflavin (Vitamin B_2)

Again one of the richest sources of this vitamin is wheat-germ, and another source is yeast. It has a similar effect to that of vitamin B_1 in the oxidisation of carbohydrates, as well as playing an important part in the health of certain types of epithelial tissue.

Niacin (Vitamin B_3)

This vitamin is also known as nicotinic acid. It is present in yeast associations, nuts, fish and meat. Niacin helps to form enzymes which aid the assimilation of carbohydrates and is a necessary catalyst for the functioning of vitamins B_1 and B_2.

Choline

Another member of the B complex, choline is present in most of the foods mentioned previously in this group. Its total action is difficult to define other than that its presence is essential for the total action of the vitamin B group. It is also suggested that choline has an effect upon the digestion, transportation and deposition of fats.

Pyridoxine (Vitamin B$_6$)

The source of pyridoxine is identical to those of the vitamins of this group previously mentioned. It is essential for the correct action of vitamins B$_1$ and B$_2$ as well as playing an important part in the nitrogen balance of the body.

Vitamin B$_{12}$

As far as sport is concerned this is the vogue vitamin. It is the only member of the vitamin B complex not found in yeast products. However, meat and dairy products have a high yield. Its original association was with anaemia, particularly pernicious anaemia, a failing of the red blood cell-producing mechanism in the bone marrow. More recently this vitamin has been associated with the cellular metabolism of carbohydrates.

Other members of the vitamin B complex include pantothenic acid, biotin, para-amino-benzoic acid and inositol. They are all present in yeast products and work closely with the other members of the vitamin B group to produce healthy life.

Vitamin C (Ascorbic Acid)

This is certainly the vitamin about which the majority of people have most knowledge, albeit a superficial knowledge usually gleaned from advertisements or literature associated with fruit, fruit drinks, protection from common colds, etc. It is certainly available in all forms of citrus fruits and most fresh green vegetables. However, its action in the body is a little more complicated than just preventing viral infections such as colds.

Its action is closely associated with the absorption of iron, an essential pigment for the transportation of oxygen, and directly for the carrying of hydrogen. It is also necessary for the health of all connective tissues including cartilage, ligaments and veins. Cooking, storing and preserving considerably reduces the levels of vitamin C in any food.

Vitamin D

This is a group composed mainly of Vitamin D$_2$ (ergosterol), which has a vegetable source, calciferol, the 'sunlight vitamin', and Vitamin D$_3$, which comes from an animal source. Its main function in health is to aid the production of strong bones and teeth. In fact, the disease of rickets has been almost completely eliminated due to a better understanding of nutritional health. All mothers will be only too familiar with the various forms of fish oils, a rich source of Vitamin D, and/or A, C, and D vitamin drops which they conscientiously feed to their offspring.

Vitamin E (Tocopherol)

This vitamin is known to exist in several forms which have been given a Greek alphabet nomenclature – alphatocopherol, beta-tocopherol, etc. In recent years this group of vitamins has attracted considerable attention because of its believed connection with fertility. Apart from this debatable function, vitamin E is known to have an effect upon the body's store of vitamin A and C, mainly through its action on the digestive tract and upon the well-being of skeletal muscle tissue. Vitamin E is present in most seed oils.

There are other known vitamins such as vitamin K, which is said to have an effect upon blood and blood vessels, and vitamin P, the bioflavonoids which are similar to vitamin C.

Recently the manufacturers of vitamin supplements have bombarded the public with advertising literature giving the whole topic a position of false importance.

Minerals

Many people confuse the presence and action of minerals with those of vitamins. While their total effect upon healthy life might be similar, their action is entirely different.

Basically the mineral action in the body can be divided into two groups: those minerals which are essential for the delicate fluid/salt balance, including sodium, potassium and chloride; and the other essential minerals, which include calcium, phosphor, magnesium, zinc and iron.

Calcium is essential for bone structure and its presence is necessary for the correct rhythmical function of cardiac and associated circulatory tissue. It is also associated with the normal assimilation of phosphor and protein. Calcium can be stored in the body in a number of ways, particularly in the gut, as a 'soap' binding with excess fats. The main sources of this mineral are dairy products and green vegetables.

Phosphor, together with magnesia, is essential for the correct functioning of nervous and muscle tissue. Magnesium combines with both calcium and phosphor in the growth and repair of bone tissue. Zinc is an essential element in insulin and in the enzymes which aid protein synthesis.

Iron is the essential element in haemoglobin, which is the oxygen-carrying pigment of the blood. This is an essential mineral as there is no place for the anaemic in high-level sport. However, this aspect will be discussed fully later in the book.

In addition to these minerals, there are other trace elements which are essential to health. These include chromium, nickel, tin, vanadium, silicon and fluoride. Their precise action is not fully understood, with the world's researchers producing daily fresh evidence which is beyond the scope of this text.

Fluid/electrolyte balance

As mentioned earlier, most of the digestive enzymes, minerals and electrolytes are carried by water. Each day about 10 litres (over 2 gallons) of water enters the alimentary canal; of this 10 litres over 90 per cent has been absorbed by the time the digestive process is complete. In bouts of high activity, water is also lost through sweat. It is essential for healthy life for the fluid balance to be kept and the body must take sufficient through drink, and absorbed in food, to keep this balance.

Dietary fibre

As well as the nutrients, which are absorbed through our digestive system, the diet also contains plant material which is not digested or absorbed in any way from the intestine. This vegetable material is frequently known as roughage. One might ask what its place is in the diet, since it passes through the system unchanged by the process of digestion. Its action is almost certainly twofold. Fibres can absorb bile acids, which are necessary for digestion but can ultimately have a bad effect upon the health of the intestine, particularly on cholesterol metabolism. The same fibres considerably increase the water content of the stools, so acting as a diluent of materials in the colon which are likely to have an adverse side-effect on the surrounding tissue composing the lower end of the digestive tract. It is a well-established fact that the incidence of illness of the lower intestine is considerably less in countries where the diet contains a high percentage of vegetable fibre.

The aim of this chapter has been to present a layman's understanding of the biological and biochemical sciences involved in nutrition. It is hoped that sufficient background information has been provided to enable the reader to understand the rest of the text fully without reference to other works.

2

Energy and energy systems

The pure physicist recognises energy as the capacity to do work. It exists in many different forms, each with the potential to be converted from one form to another. All of the energy used by man is ultimately derived from the sun, where it exists in the form of radiant energy. While animals cannot use solar energy directly, they do so indirectly via the food which they eat. The plant converts radiant energy to chemical energy by the process known as photosynthesis. Here the action of sunlight, together with chlorophyl (the green pigment in plants), converts atmospheric carbon dioxide to carbohydrates. It is the job of the food producer to concentrate this form of energy into substances which can fulfil man's nutritional needs. This can be done directly, by growing cereal crops, or plants which store starch in their roots (e.g. potatoes) or indirectly through animals and their products. Man is not provided with the ability to take direct advantage of green plants as a potential energy store. Animals, which have a different alimentary canal, can digest the cellulose in the plants and convert it to a chemical energy to build their tissue, which in turn man consumes.

So, in basic terms, the nutritionist is concerned with radiant energy, which man converts to chemical energy, thus providing a potential to convert to mechanical and heat energy. Because energy can be converted from one form to another each can be measured in units applicable to that particular form of energy. For example, when mechanical energy is considered the units used are related to work, so involving the units of force and distance. These include the dyne and newton (force); centimetre and metre (distance); and erg and joule (work) – see below. However, the nutritionist uses a unit based on a heat measurement, that is, the calorie. But for convenience the unit is further modified into the kilocalorie or Calorie, i.e. one thousand calories. For example, the human body at rest utilises energy at the rate of 1 Calorie per minute. The output of a 1-kilowatt electric fire is about 14 Cal/min, so it is easy to see why one feels hot in a small, crowded room.

Units of force, energy and power

1 **dyne**	the force required to accelerate 1 g 1 cm/sec/sec
1 **newton**	the force required to accelerate 1 kg 1 m/sec/sec
1 **erg**	the work performed when a force of 1 dyne moves through 1 cm
1 **joule**	the work performed when a force of 1 newton moves through 1 m 1 joule = 2.38×10^{-1} calories
1 **calorie**	the heat required to raise the temperature of 1 g water 1 ^{0}C. 1 calorie = 4.1868 joules. 1000 calories = 1 Calorie
1 **watt**	the power equal to a rate of working of 1 joule/sec or 2.388×10^{-1} cals/sec.

Energy content in food

When the human body converts the chemical energy in foods it does so through an oxidative process only made possible by enzymes. In other words, without the enzymes the energy in foods could not be released through combustion at body temperature. If the foods are completely burnt in a special process involving oxygen at a high pressure, the heat given out in the combustion process can be measured in Calories, so giving a particular type of food a calorific value. The apparatus used for operating this forced combustion is known as the bomb calorimeter. In this process a particular food is mixed with oxygen at high pressure, ignited by an electric spark and the heat liberated by the combustion is accurately measured. Using the calorimetry technique it can be calculated that each gram of carbohydrate has an energy potential of 4.1 Cal/g, protein about 5.6 Cal/g and fats in the region of 9.3 Cal/g.

However, these figures cannot be used directly in calculations dealing with the animal conversion of the foods. This is because the human digestive process is not as complete as the bomb calorimeter. The human body cannot fully digest all foods and extract the total energy potential, so some is excreted in the faeces. Also, breakdown of the foodstuff at tissue level is never complete, especially with proteins, so Calories are lost or excreted in the urine. The human digestive system is over 90 per cent efficient, this value varying according to the type of food; the lowest percentage is for protein, where about 8 per cent is lost, representing about 1.25 Cal/g, and the highest is for carbohydrates, where the system is about 99 per cent efficient. So, as far as the human body is concerned, each gram of carbohydrate yields about 4 Cal, each gram of protein about 4 Cal and each gram of fats about 9 Cal.

Most texts on nutrition list tables of food and their energy equivalents. In most cases these have been calculated through analysis which approximately breaks down a particular food into the major categories of protein, fat, carbohydrate and water; the formula listed above, that is that 1 g of protein yields 4 Cal, etc., is then applied. While these tables cannot be precise, they serve as a very valuable guide. If precision is required, then extra allowance must be made for absorption losses and the carbohydrates group would need to be broken down into monosaccharides and polysaccharides. Even with these allowances it must be accepted that different food samples vary slightly in their chemical composition, so making it extremely difficult for this to be an exact science. Even so, most food tables calculated in this way can be regarded as 85–90 per cent accurate, so making them sufficient for practical purposes. Table 1 illustrates some of the common foods in our diet together with a total energy equivalent and the breakdown into major components. The value is per 100 grams of the food.

Table 1 *Common foods, showing energy equivalents and major food components*

	Energy Cal	Water g	Protein g	Fats g	Carbo-hydrates g
bread	243	38.3	7.8	1.4	52.7
milk	66	87.0	3.4	3.7	4.8
butter	793	13.9	0.4	85.1	Slight
cheese	425	37.0	25.4	34.5	Slight
potatoes (raw)	70	80.0	2.5	Slight	15.9
cabbage (raw)	20	78.0	1.3	Slight	1.3
peas (cooked)	80	72.0	6.0	Slight	16.0
meat	270	56.0	20.0	20.0	0
fish	17.5	65.0	20.0	8.3	3.6
apple	47	84.1	0.3	Slight	12.2
bananas	60	60.0	0.7	Slight	14.0
tomatoes	20	75.0	1.0	Slight	5.8
cucumber	15	80.0	0.5	Slight	5.2

Energy balance

Energy degradation is a necessary part of life. While its rate varies considerably between individuals and from moment to moment, it never ceases during life. Energy turnover at complete rest is at a minimum or basal level. It is at its maximum during physical exertion and can approach more than twenty times the basal level. While work does have an effect upon energy expenditure, this effect is not as great as most people would think. This is because the muscles are only active in this way for a short period of time compared with the total day or year.

In very basic terms, an individual must take in, through food, sufficient energy to balance that used in total life. If the input exceeds the output then the energy is stored about the body in the form of fat. If the input is less than the output, the body is in a katabolic state and will ultimately break down. If the input far exceeds the output, the fat store becomes excessive and the individual is obese. While the energy balance of an individual changes very little over a day, its accumulative effect over a period of years can be considerable. An extra slice of bread and butter makes no significant difference to the daily energy balance, yet over a period of fifty years the accumulative effect could be very significant. During maturity the average person gains about 12 kg (26 lb) in weight yet eats in excess of 20,000 kg (20 tons) of food. This weight gain represents an excess intake of food over energy requirements of 350 mg (0.01 oz) per day, something well short of the value of an extra portion of bread and butter.

Hence, for healthy life over the adult cycle it is necessary for this energy balance to be maintained.

The average person has an energy requirement of about 3,000 Cals per day. It must be emphasised that this is an average figure because it is proportional to bodyweight and the basic metabolism of the individual, as well as the degree of activity.

In 1961 the National Food Survey Committee published the following figures to show the average amount of energy which was available per day for each resident in the United Kingdom. As can be seen, it provides an energy equivalent of 3,170 Cals. I would suggest that while the energy requirement of the average person is less now than it was in 1961, it is doubtful whether the associated comparative reduction in food has taken place.

Table 2 *Amounts of energy available per person per day*

	g	energy Cal	% of total energy
Protein	68	350	11
Fat	141	1,230	39
Carbohydrate	414	1,590	50
Total energy		3,170	

Table 2 indicates that, as far as energy is concerned, only 11 per cent of the total requirement needs to be in the form of protein, and by far the greatest proportion comes from carbohydrates.

Energy expenditure

While it is possible to calculate, in terms of external work, the amount of energy physically used in its execution, this would only represent part of the total expenditure, since it would not take into account the energy used in internal work (movement of heart, respiratory muscles, etc.). The total calculation of energy expenditure is made possible by the principle that *all* energy used in the body is converted to heat. If the total output of heat can be measured, then this can be converted to the total energy used in its production.

Research workers have two methods open to them for determining energy expenditure – direct and indirect calorimetry. The direct method involves the use of a special room with sensitive temperature-measuring devices and methods for monitoring inspired and expired air. The subject sleeps, eats and performs functions of work inside the chamber. Results of experiments using the indirect calorimetry method established that humans obey the first law of thermodynamics in that the energy available in the food eaten by a person exactly equals the energy lost in heat. The researchers also established that the energy calculated from the oxygen consumption was equal to the measured heat output. This proved that the computations used with the direct method validated those obtained from the indirect method, so making experiments on energy expenditure simpler and less costly as they avoided the use of the human calorimeter.

The indirect calorimetry technique involves the measurement of the inspired and expired air and the calculation of oxygen utilisation and carbon dioxide production. Energy is derived from the oxidisation of foodstuffs; in the process oxygen is used and carbon dioxide liberated. The ratio of carbon dioxide to oxygen, CO_2/O_2, is known as the respiratory quotient (RQ). Each of the food categories has a different RQ because of their different chemical structure. For example, carbohydrates have an RQ of 1. In the carbohydrate molecule the proportion of hydrogen and oxygen is the same as in water. Hence, during oxidisation oxygen is required for the oxidisation of both hydrogen and carbon. When a fat is oxidised, oxygen is required for the oxidisation of both hydrogen and carbon so more oxygen is used, decreasing its respiratory quotient. See below.

Table 3 *Respiratory quotients*

	Respiratory quotient	Litres O_2 required	Litres CO_2 produced
1 g carbohydrate	1.0	0.828	0.828
(starch)	0.7	2.019	1.427
1 g fat (animal)	approx. 0.8	0.961	0.781

The precise value for protein is difficult to measure because of its variable source. However, energy is seldom derived from the oxidisation of protein, since it is the last in the chain, with stores of carbohydrate and fat being sufficient to cope even in quite extreme situations. Experiments on energy expenditure can tell whether protein is used as a source of energy since nitrogen is deposited in the urine proportional to the amount of protein oxidised. Knowing this, it is simple to calculate the amount of fats and carbohydrates oxidised for energy by measuring the amount of oxygen used and carbon dioxide produced and using the RQ values listed in Table 3.

The research worker has several methods open for indirect calorimetry gas sampling and gas analysis, but the methods are beyond the scope of this text. Photograph 1(a), showing an athlete exercising at the Carnegie Laboratory of the Leeds Polytechnic, illustrates one of the methods, where the gas is collected in Douglas bags.

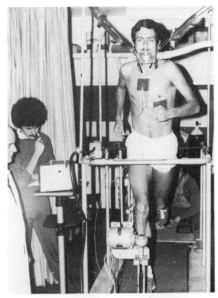

1(a) (left) *Treadmill running in the laboratory*

1(b) (below left) *Measuring skin folds is a method for calculating lean body mass or fat deposits*

1(c) (below right) *Measuring of skin folds on the upper arm using calipers*

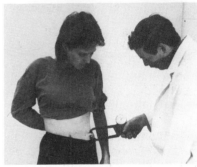

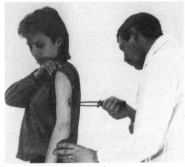

These three photographs show the ways in which the research worker can calculate the energy requirements of certain activities and the effects they are likely to have on the body

Metabolism

In simple terms there are two types of metabolism, which ultimately amount to one and the same thing. Energy metabolism is the way an individual uses the energy derived from food to perform the necessary functions of life and to do physical work. Chemical metabolism is the way the chemical energy of the nutrients from the diet is converted to chemical energy stored in the body in the form of energy-rich compounds. All cellular energy comes from the breakdown of a substance known as adenosine triphosphate (ATP). The body must always have a supply of this substance and there are several systems by which the body can ensure that there is a constant supply. In sport, we refer to them as energy systems and they will be discussed later in the text.

The liver is the 'director' of most metabolic pathways and plays a leading role in the metabolism of carbohydrates, fats and proteins. All products of digestion, absorbed from the alimentary canal into the blood, pass through the liver, where they are changed, stored or passed on unchanged. The liver is able to convert one form of amino-acid to another or convert them into carbohydrates or fatty acids. It can convert carbohydrates to fatty acids and forms plasma proteins from the amino-acids. In addition to this it serves as a detoxifying agent which neutralises some of the harmful substances absorbed during digestion or produced during metabolism.

Each of the basic nutrients (carbohydrates, fats and proteins) is metabolised in a different way. Carbohydrates are absorbed from the alimentary canal in the form of fructose, galactose or glucose and are converted in the liver and stored there as glycogen. Glycogen has to be converted in the mitochondria of the cells to ATP. The sequence of events then depends upon whether or not enough oxygen is available for the process to metabolise aerobically (with sufficient oxygen) or anaerobically (in the absence of sufficient oxygen).

In the presence of oxygen, glycogen is broken down into ATP and its by-products are pyruvic acid, carbon dioxide and water. Each molecule of glycogen yields thirty-eight molecules of ATP. In the absence of oxygen, glycogen is still oxidised but one of the by-products is lactic acid. Since the body requires ATP all the time there must be a system ensuring its continual availability. There are very many reactions, all involving coenzymes, which ensure the presence of this vital substance. Diagram 2 attempts to illustrate the process, together with the cycles which keep the supply of energy available. It must be remembered that each of the reactions involved in glycolysis, the Cori cycle (the resynthesis of lactic acid to glycogen) and the citric acid cycle (Kreb cycle) all require energy. The citric acid cycle only takes place in the presence of oxygen, so it is part of aerobic metabolism. It takes place in the mitochondria of the cell where, under the action of enzymes, adenosine diphosphate (ADP, the by-product when energy is liberated from ATP) is reconstituted as ATP. The important catalyst in this reaction is coenzyme A which reacts with pyruvic acid to form acetyl coenzyme A. Acetyl coenzyme A is also derived from the metabolism of fatty acids and some amino-acids. Hence, the metabolism of fats for energy joins the citric acid cycle when they are broken down into units of acetyl coenzyme A and are then metabolised as carbohydrates.

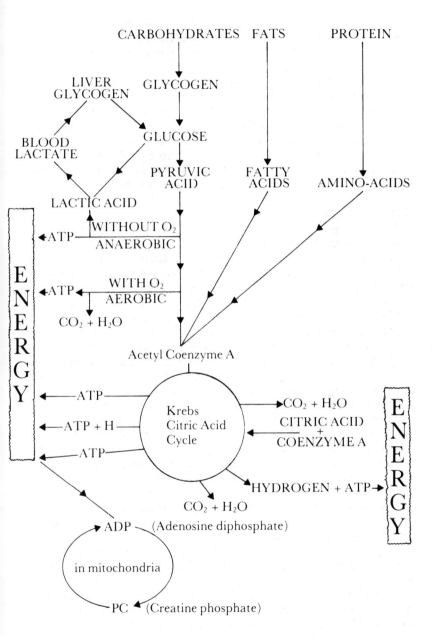

Diagram 2 illustrates the means by which the body produces energy from food

Normally the body does not derive energy from the breakdown of proteins. When proteins are metabolised the amino-acids are converted to keto acids and form ammonia. The keto acids are then converted to acetyl coenzyme A and join the citric acid cycle to be metabolised as carbohydrates. As the ammonia is toxic it is converted in the liver to urea, which is excreted.

Energy systems

Energy for violent physical exercise is required instantly before the blood supply can provide an adequate supply of oxygen to permit the complete oxidisation of glucose. Hence all early activity is anaerobic and relies upon the store of glycogen which the muscle cells have. The following is a brief synopsis of the levels, which can be related to diagram 2.

First level
Glycogen stored in the muscle cells is converted to ATP. This is sufficient for about three seconds of exercise and the by-product is ADP.

Second level
The cells have a store of creatine phosphate which can be used to reconstitute ATP. This store again is sufficient for about three seconds of exercise.

Third level
After this short period of time the system must rely upon glycogen stored in the liver. When ATP is broken down to form ADP, pyruvic acid is produced. This is converted to lactic acid, some of which enters the Cori cycle and is reconstituted in the liver to form liver glycogen. See diagram 2.

Nowadays coaches, particularly in the sport of track and field athletics, pay considerable attention to these energy systems since it is their belief that each system responds differently to the various forms of training.

3

Special considerations

The previous chapter served as a brief introduction to energy and energy metabolism. However, one's metabolic rate is not constant. It varies with age, size, climate, degree of activity, etc. Even the basal (resting) metabolic rate varies from person to person and is controlled by the secretion of hormones, an aspect beyond the scope of this book. The other factors can be discussed, since they are of interest to those involved in the nutrition of sportsmen and women.

Effect of size

This is an important factor and one frequently ignored when considering the nutritional requirements for, in particular, big field-event performers. In the previous chapter energy was linked to work, which, by physical definition, is the product of the force and the range through which the force acts. Let us compare the simple work performed by two people, person A weighing 10 stone and person B weighing 15 stone, each stepping up a stair 1 foot high. For simplicity, I will use the units of foot-pounds to make the comparison. The force in each case is that required to overcome the pull of gravity.

Work performed by person A – 140 x 1 = 140 ft lb
Work performed by person B – 210 x 1 = 210 ft lb

Ignoring any time factor, it follows that in this simple comparison of work the equivalent energy expenditure is proportional to the mass. That is, a 50 per cent increase in body weight gives a 50 per cent increase in work output. This factor also helps to illustrate the extra strain which could be placed on a system through overweight, a factor which is constantly the concern of those associated with energy balance.

Effect of age

In experiments involving young children it was found that, as far as metabolism is concerned, bodyweight is a more critical factor than age. However, with adolescents both age and sex become considered factors. D. F. Talbot (USA) in a paper published in 1938, *Basal*

Metabolism Standards for Children, indicated that the metabolic rate per unit of weight falls with age. In comparing a 3 kg (6.6 lb) baby, a 30 kg (66 lb) child, a 60 kg (132 lb) adolescent boy and a 65 kg (143 lb) adult man, he found that resting metabolic rates are 34, 26, 19 and 17 Cal/min/kg respectively. It must be remembered that these are average figures for the basal rate. With exercise both would increase proportionally. But it does illustrate that even at basal rates the energy requirements of young children are higher than for adults.

With increasing age, the important factor is the reduction in physical activity. This is associated with the reduced ability of the heart and lungs to supply the working muscles with oxygen and nutrients.

Effect of climate

The fact that most people find that their appetite increases while they are on holiday at the seaside, or working out of doors on cold days, and that it decreases on very hot days, is nature's indication that climate does affect metabolism. However, it is not just air temperature which affects metabolism. It is affected equally by humidity, composition of the atmosphere and the amount of air movement. When a person moves from one type of climate to another a period of acclimatisation is necessary before the metabolism adjusts to the change. In some cases the acclimatisation is complete, in others it is only partial. This illustrates that heredity plays a significant role and that the immigrant's adaptation can never make him as completely suited to his environment as the native. A classic example is adaptation to altitude, a problem which was brought home to the world of sport when the Olympic Games were held in 1968 in Mexico City, at an elevation of 2,200 m (7,200 ft).

In extremes of temperature it is difficult to decide whether the obvious change in the metabolic rate is directly due to the environment or whether it is due to the change in levels of activity. For example, in very cold climates protective clothing is necessary, which imposes restrictions on movement, so increasing the energy cost for a particular activity. Researchers have found that activity in a very hot environment increases the oxygen consumption by about 10 per cent compared with the same activity in a cooler situation.

Top-level sport now takes the competitor to all the extremes of environment. If the competition is to be on equal terms then due consideration must be paid to the changes in nutritional requirements forced by the environment, and the necessary period allowed for acclimatisation to the new environment.

Effect of sport

As outlined earlier, the energy requirements are directly related to the physical output in terms of work. While it is not the brief of this text to consider the energy expenditure required by one's occupation, it is of considerable interest in the total situation. This will be dealt with fully when the special requirements for sport are considered. It is obvious that the manual worker expends more energy in the course of his occupation than does the more sedentary office worker. While it must be accepted that mechanisation has reduced this difference considerably, the energy gap between the extremes of occupation is still a large factor.

This situation always prompts stimulating discussion on whether sportsmen are best recruited from manual or sedentary occupations. The manual worker, just in the course of performing his occupation, develops the 'physiological system' that could be advantageous to sport. Yet at the end of the day he is often too tired to perform the specific training necessary to participate. The sedentary worker can tackle a training programme with enthusiasm at the end of the day because of the contrast between his occupation and leisure. The discussion will always continue, but one thing is certain: it is no longer possible to work physically hard during the day and then expect to develop the expertise necessary to compete at top level. So, while recruitment from manual workers is often desirable, top-level sport will certainly force a change in occupation.

As a society changes and becomes more prosperous, the demand for recreation and leisure time increases. Nowadays, most men and women are more physically active in their non-occupational activities than they are in their salaried job of work. As far as I am concerned this change is essential for the continued health of society. With the reduction in manual work, the ease of transport, etc. on one side, and the increased wealth, providing greater opportunity for over-indulging in eating, drinking, smoking and other habit-forming (yet detrimental to health) pastimes on the other, it becomes essential for society to establish a balance in an attempt to prevent man from following a course of self-destruction. Many people will be able to cite examples of longevity associated with inactivity, and of sportspeople who have died young. There are always exceptions to any rule. But the therapeutic effect of exercise in the prevention of obesity and cardiac complaints is beyond dispute. Hence society must plan for, and direct, this essential aspect of community life.

The amount of energy used in recreation varies considerably from sport to sport and from person to person within the same sport. For example, the amount of energy expended in a game of bowls is unlikely to be the same as that used in a strenuous cross-country run. A number of research workers have tried to classify recreational activities according to their energy demands. For example, according to Durnin and Passmore in *Energy, Work and Leisure* (1967), archery, bowls, cricket, sailing and table-tennis are listed as 'light' activities, badminton, canoeing, gymnastics, hockey, tennis and swimming as 'moderate', and athletics, basketball, climbing, football, rowing and squash have 'heavy' rankings. While I accept this in very broad, general terms it does not take into account the levels of performance. For example, to swim (moderate rating with Durnin/Passmore) 100 metres in 60 seconds is certainly more demanding in energy than to run ('heavy' activity) 400 metres in 60 seconds. Of course, this introduces the argument of specificity and skill levels, which are very positive considerations. This topic will be more fully dealt with later.

It has only been the intention of this chapter to introduce the special considerations which have an effect upon metabolism and energy requirements. However, it must be emphasised that the secretion of hormones affecting the body chemistry has a far greater effect upon metabolism than any extrinsic factors such as environment and exercise. In this chapter, I have often made reference to 'man'; in all cases one could equally substitute 'woman'. However, there is a definite sex difference in metabolism which can be related to hormone secretion and body chemistry, particularly, for example, during pregnancy.

4
Diet fads and fallacies

It is not the intention of this chapter to condemn outright any of the particular fads which those associated with sport have. Rather the aim is to give scientific support, or rejection, to some of the common fads and fallacies. At the same time I obviously recognise that the razor's edge of defeat or victory is set not by physiological but by the psychological fads (see p. 93). If, for example, an athlete has established a particular whim which has some psychological foundation it might be that the psychological advantage outweighs the physiological disadvantage. At times, it almost suggests a study of black magic, for which I am not qualified. It is also unfortunate that certain manufacturing and marketing agencies cash in on this trait and make handsome profits from those striving for sporting excellence. Many of the fads come and go and remain the vogue only as long as a particular champion acclaims their success, or until another champion comes along extolling a different 'open sesame' to fame. Other fads are like old wives' tales; no one knows their exact origin, but they are handed down from generation to generation and, like the fisherman's tale, become more exaggerated with the passing of time.

Probably the most hallowed of the time-honoured fads is the need for the pre-match steak or even the large emphasis on beefsteak in the diet for sportspeople. Certainly, as a pre-match meal, this must be refuted. Steak has a very slow transit time through the digestive tract, taking up to four hours or more to complete the process. Should the body need to use the proteins for energy they have to be converted to carbohydrates. This process involves a reaction, the by-product of which is urea, a toxin that has to be removed from the body. Exercise produces similar toxins, thus making the combined effect of the removal of waste products excessive, placing an unnecessary strain on the excretory mechanism.

During exercise the splanchnic (gut) area of the body is partially deprived of blood. A total supply of blood is necessary for the complete digestion of foods, together with the removal of waste products. It is, therefore, important to have the digestive system relatively inactive during exercise. This certainly would not be the case with a pre-event meal containing steak, unless, that is, the exercise time is delayed by at least four hours. With this in mind it can be established that the pre-event meal should be one which is quickly digested and contains a relatively high energy content. However, this will be fully discussed in Chapter 8.

Society is made conscious that the body needs protein as it is vital to life and can only be obtained from the food eaten. This situation then tends to foster the philosophy that because something is good more of the same has to be better. While this is a very simple philosophy, there is little evidence to support it as far as nutrition is concerned. Society tends to justify what it likes doing, and this certainly seems to be the case as far as animal protein is concerned. The slow transit time of this type of food through the gut produces a 'satisfied' feeling with an associated euphoric effect. It is fairly certain that this fad develops from the euphoria. Of course the body needs protein, but an excess is merely converted to carbohydrates and used to provide energy or to be distributed about the body as fatty tissue. Animal protein is one of the most expensive foods so this particular fad could prove very costly.

One has only to spend a short while in the company of field events athletes to realise that many have an obsession for drinking milk. It is not uncommon to find athletes whose daily intake of this beverage is in excess of 6 litres (10 pints). Again, this is a fad which is difficult to understand. It has been suggested, by several authorities, that milk is one of the most complete foods. As far as human beings are concerned, there is no such thing as the complete food. However, it is likely that opinion could be formed and influenced by the fact that the early life of all mammals is supported entirely by milk. The milk most commonly used for human consumption is cow's milk, which has a completely different amino-acid balance from that which is required by the human body. Hence, it must be appreciated that milk is not a complete food.

Milk also has a high fat and calcium content. In excessive milk drinkers it is possible that it could help the diet to contain too much of these two elements. While they are not directly toxic, neither, in excess, contributes to good health.

A fad which has recently crept in, mainly through high-pressure advertising, is the use of glucose tablets or drinks before competition. Some manufacturing companies offer pseudo-research data to back up their product, suggesting that controlled experiments have been performed to support its benefit, particularly for endurance sports.

It is true that for sports lasting in excess of ten minutes, blood sugar levels must be kept constant. The problem with ingestion of high levels of glucose is controlling the level. It is possible to produce a situation of hyperglycemia where the blood sugar levels remain high for a period of time, which might aid performance. However, such an effect is likely to be short-lived because of the insulin reaction. Nature is very sensitive to any change in its homeostatic state. Should the balance be disturbed, nature takes regressive steps to return it to a level with which it is familiar. In the case of blood sugar levels, this balance is kept with the flow of insulin. Hence, if the insulin reaction is triggered off it is possible to get an 'over-shoot' so that the body ends up with a lower blood sugar level than before the ingestion.

It is most difficult to suggest hard and fast rules, because the situation varies from individual to individual. It might be possible to justify the taking of glucose products on psychological grounds but their effect would be difficult to prove on any other plane.

With the ever-improving levels of performance in sport, participants will explore every avenue open to them to enhance their performances. Such a route which is both explored and exploited is that of vitamins. As explained earlier, the field of vitamins represents a massive area of study with new, or supposedly new, vitamins being found yearly. The indiscriminate use of vitamins can prove both costly and harmful: costly in that many are not required and are merely excreted, and harmful in that certain vitamins, taken in excess, are toxic. However, having said this, I am of the opinion that vitamin therapy, for certain classes of sportsmen and women, is worthwhile. Specific details of this will be given in Chapters 6 and 7.

Because the study of vitamins is a very specialised area, and in some cases the precise action of vitamins is not fully understood, commercial exploitation is facilitated. The human body, in a 'low' state, is susceptible to any proposed pick-me-up whether its efficacy is in doubt or not. For every study supporting vitamin therapy in the remedial field, there is one contradicting its value. Thus an atmosphere of uncertainty is created, and as long as this doubt remains, the athlete becomes gullible and open to the rich pickings of the unethical element of the nutritional field.

Many sportspeople feel that there is a need to eat extra salt because the activity of sport increases the rate of heat lost through sweating and the associated loss of body salt. It is true that the body does lose salt through perspiration, but it is not the loss of salt that is dangerous to the body but rather the upsetting of the electrolyte balance. It has been estimated that the normal person requires about 5 grams ($\frac{1}{6}$ oz) of salt per day and that the average intake is in the region of 10–15 grams ($\frac{1}{3}$-$\frac{1}{2}$ oz), that is, about twice as much as is really required. Rather than consider the amount of salt taken per day in isolation it would seem more logical to consider it in the context of the amount of fluid lost and that required to replace it to prevent dehydration. Experts in the field suggest that an extra gram of salt per litre of fluid (0.02 oz per pint) is more than sufficient to redress the balance. If excessive salt is taken this can contribute to dehydration, a condition which is far more serious than salt depletion. It has also been shown that there is a significant correlation between high blood pressure and people who use excessive amounts of salt in their diet.

It is quite obvious that extra salt is not required by the majority of sportspeople unless they are exercising in very hot, humid conditions. In these conditions, there is value in using one of the common salt tablets to aid the performer through a period of acclimatisation. Once the period of acclimatisation is passed, which can take two or three weeks, the perspiration gradually starts to contain less salt and the need for any extra dietary intake is lost.

5

Exercise metabolism

As mentioned earlier, a balance must exist between the total energy expenditure and the energy equivalent of the food intake. If the energy expenditure exceeds that of intake then a katabolic (breakdown) process takes place, which will ultimately result in death. If the energy equivalent of the food exceeds the total energy output then fatty tissue is formed.

The sportsperson who expends more energy than the average person must take in more food to allow for the level of activity. The amount of food required by the sportsperson can now be calculated with some degree of accuracy. The considerations are:
1. basal metabolic rate
2. the energy cost of the work involved in performing the usual daily functions of life
3. the energy cost of the sporting activity performed.

If these three are added together a reasonable figure for total energy requirement should be reached. Age also has an effect, with a negative differential of 4 per cent for each decade above twenty-five years old.

1. Basic metabolic rate

The basal energy requirement is the calories expended in twenty-four hours of complete bed-rest. It is dependent upon sex, height and weight. For example, it has been found that a 64 kg (140 lb) man has a Calorie expenditure of 1,550 Calories while a 64 kg woman has an expenditure of 1,400 Calories. The following list gives the approximate basal energy expenditure for the various weight classifications.

Men		
Weight		*Calorie expenditure*
140 lb	(64 kg)	1,550
160 lb	(73 kg)	1,640
180 lb	(82 kg)	1,730
200 lb	(91 kg)	1,815
220 lb	(100 kg)	1,900
Women		
Weight		*Calorie expenditure*
100 lb	(45 kg)	1,225
120 lb	(54 kg)	1,320
140 lb	(64 kg)	1,400
160 lb	(73 kg)	1,485
180 lb	(82 kg)	1,575

These calculations are based on a man whose height is 5 ft 10 in (178 cm). If taller than this standard, 20 Calories per inch (25 mm) should be added to the total. If shorter, 20 Calories per inch should be subtracted. In the case of women, the standard height is 5 ft 6 in (168 cm) with the same caloric differentials.

2. Energy costs of normal daily functions

These must be added to the basal requirements to calculate the energy costs of normal daily life.

Activity	Calories/kg/hour
Sitting still	1.43
Standing	1.50
Walking	2.86
Dressing/undressing	1.69
Light work (typing)	2.00
Moderate work	5.70
Heavy occupational work	7.50

Appendix A will list a more detailed breakdown for a wider variety of activities. With these figures it is possible to calculate an approximate percentage differential above the basal rate:

Activity	Above basal
Quiet sitting	30%
Light activity (office work)	50%
Moderate activity	70%
Heavy occupational activity	100%

For example, a 45-year-old man, 5 ft 10 in (178 cm), weighing 200 lb (91 kg) and involved in heavy manual work has a total energy requirement as follows:

Basal rate	1815	
Manual work 100%	1815	
	3630	
Less 8% for age differential	290	
	3340	Calories per day

3. Energy cost of sport

Because of the various levels of participation, it is difficult to arrive at a precise figure for the energy cost of a particular sport. It becomes easier to calculate when the sport is speed-related, such as walking, running and swimming a set distance. When it is considered that sport embraces activities ranging from comparatively sedate sports like archery and bowls to such energetic sports as marathon running and rugby football, it is obvious that there will be a considerable variation in energy expenditure, hence the grading tables by Durnin and Passmore, listed on p. 30.

The level of participation is a most difficult one to consider when making calculations, particularly the major team games such as rugby and Association football or hockey. For calculations to approach a degree of accuracy in these games it would be necessary to do a player/positional analysis of a 'typical' game. In such an analysis it would be possible to log the total distance run and the total time taken, the degree of body contact, the number of strikes, kicks or throws, etc., and from this calculate the energy expenditure. It is fairly certain that the directors of coaching in these sports will have this level of information available.

Skill

There is a saying that the skilled performer always makes a task look effortless. The statement is, broadly speaking, correct; but only by comparison. The efforts of the novice certainly look clumsy when compared with a skilled performer. However, the contrast is not so apparent when two people of equal ability are compared. The skilled performer eliminates unnecessary movements and so in this respect conserves energy. This effect is probably most marked in swimming, where a poor stroke has a retarding effect and is, therefore, wasteful in terms of energy. The same might also be said of running events, where the relaxed runner can save a considerable amount of energy, especially in those events of a sustained nature. However, while it is obviously possible to recognise skill levels, it is a factor which is most difficult to allow for when making calculations relating to energy expenditure, especially when it is a subjective assessment of skill that is being made. The idea of looking carefully into the nutrition of sportspeople is just one of the avenues one must explore in the pursuit of excellence. It could be that little extra that might be sufficient to tip the scales in one's favour. In this respect, the unskilled performer is not a consideration and the view held by most dieticians that for the average person, a normal diet is quite adequate, certainly holds true.

The list on the next page, compiled from information given by Sharkey in *Physiology and Physical Activity* and by Yakovlev in *Nutrition of the Athlete*, gives most sports together with a calorific energy expenditure per minute. The values given are for an average bodyweight of 68 kg (150 lb). Ten per cent should be added to this value for each 7 kg over the standard weight and 10 per cent subtracted for the same interval under the standard.

With the intermittent sports, the time spent on recovery between bouts of activity must be treated as standing or walking and calculated with the values listed on p. 94.

It would be a massive task to carry out the necessary research work to compile a table for all of the known sports. Hence, those listed are the ones commonly practised. It is possible to calculate the energy requirements of a sport not included in this list by selecting one of a related nature, or composed of a number of the sports listed.

Activity	Calories/min
Archery	5.2
Badminton (competition)	10.0
Basketball	6.0–9.0
Boxing (amateur)	10.0–15.0
Cycling 5–15 mph	5.0–12.0
Calisthenics	5.0
Judo/Karate	13.0
Rowing (vigorous)	15.0
Soccer activity	9.0
Skating (competition)	10.0
Squash	10.0
Swimming 60 m/min	29.24
Swimming 70 m/min	35.13
Tennis (competition)	11.00
Track and field athletics:	
Running 100m	51.00
Running 400 m/min	92.0
Running 5 min mile	25.0
Hurdling	21.3
Jumping	7.0
Throwing	12.46
Walking 8 km/hr	11.33
Wrestling	14.4

Further to this list, Yakovlev suggests a possible breakdown of the diet, in terms of the basic nutrients, for certain sports (see Table 4). The values listed are in grams and relate to each kilogram of bodyweight.

The calculations used to help compute the table assume that both 1 gram of protein and 1 gram of carbohydrate yield 4.1 Calories while 1 gram of fat yields 9.3 Calories.

With the aid of the various tables listed in this chapter it should be possible to establish, with some degree of accuracy, the Calorie requirement of sportspeople involved not only in the practice of their event but also in the act of carrying out the energy-demanding activities of daily life. It is the usual practice to add 10 per cent to the total calculations to allow for any inaccuracies, particularly those involved in timing.

Table 4 *Calorie content of daily diet per kg of bodyweight for different types of sport*

	Protein g/kg	Fats g/kg	Carbo-hydrate g/kg	Calories
Basketball	2.1–2.5	1.7–1.8	9.0–10.0	62–64
Boxing	2.4–2.5	2.0–2.1	9.0–10.0	65–70
Cycling (sprint)	2.1–2.3	1.9–2.0	10.0–11.0	67–73
Cycling (distance)	2.6–2.8	2.3–2.4	11.0–13.0	80–87
Football (Association)	2.3–2.4	1.8–1.9	9.0–16.0	63–67
Fencing	2.0–2.3	1.5–1.6	9.0–10.0	60–65
Gymnastics	2.1–2.3	1.5–1.6	9.5–9.6	60–65
Horseriding	2.1–2.3	2.1–2.3	8.0–9.0	61–67
Swimming	2.1–2.3	2.0–2.1	8.0–9.0	60–65
Skiing (distance)	2.0–2.1	2.0–2.1	9.0–9.6	64–67
Skating	2.0–2.1	2.0–2.1	9.0–9.6	64–67
Track and field:				
Running	2.4–2.5	1.7–1.8	9.5–10.0	65–70
Jumping	2.4–2.5	1.7–1.8	9.5–10.0	65–70
Throwing	2.4–2.5	1.7–1.8	9.5–10.0	65–70
Volleyball	2.1–2.3	1.7–1.8	9.0–10.0	62–64
Wrestling	2.4–2.5	2.0–2.1	9.0–10.0	65–70

The total energy requirement can be converted to equivalent quantities of the basic nutrients by using Table 4 above or by using an accepted ratio of 1 : 1 : 4 (by weight) for proteins, fats and carbohydrates and assuming that each gram of protein yields 4.1 Calories, each gram of carbohydrate 5.3 Calories and each gram of fat 9.3 Calories.

For endurance sports it is wise to reduce the previous ratio of 1 : 1 : 4 (by weight for proteins, fats and carbohydrates) to 1 : 0.8 : 4. This is to allow for the fact that more oxygen is required to metabolise fats and there is competition with the active tissues for this vital fuel. Under oxygen 'stress' the body readily assimilates carbohydrates.

In this discussion it must be recognised that the majority of protein ingested is used for tissue-building and only a relatively small proportion used for providing energy. Research work in Norway, using track and field athletics as the sample sport, established that throwers eat more than runners and jumpers. However, because throwers are, generally speaking, heavier than other athletes, the energy intake per kilogram of bodyweight is about the same. The same survey indicated that athletes obtained about 14 per cent of their energy requirements in the form of protein, about 40 per cent in the form of fats and 46 per cent in the form of carbohydrates.

Armed with the information to date in this chapter, the enthusiast should be able to prepare a basic diet, in terms of calories and basic nutrients, to make sure that this area of aid to physical performance will not be a weak link. The added confidence that the science of nutrition has been applied could also help the total confidence of a competitor, which can only enhance performance.

However, this only provides a basic foundation of nutritional science; it still remains to be translated into what a sportsman or woman actually needs to eat. The question of what an athlete should eat in order to improve his or her performance is just about as old as sport itself, with evidence of documentation regarding protein intake dating to the fifth century BC.

Nutrition must be regarded as a fairly precise science and the basic understanding which it must give is that because the athlete is involved in a greater energy expenditure than the average person, more of everything must be included in the diet.

Protein

With reference to table 4, p. 40, it can be seen that the average number of Calories per day, per kilogram, is about 65. If this figure is related to the average weight of 70 kg (154 lb) for a full-grown man, it can be calculated that the energy expenditure of the average-weight sportsman is almost 4,550 Calories. This represents about twice the energy requirement of the 'average person'. The average person requires about 1 g protein per kg bodyweight per day, so giving a total of 70 g. From table 4 it can be seen that the average amount of protein required for each sport per day is about twice the amount needed by the average person. Hence, it can be simply related back to the total energy requirements in calories.

While most reference texts on nutrition suggest that there is no need for the active sportsperson to include more protein in the diet than the average person, other research workers, for very valid reasons, do not support this viewpoint. Table 4 recommends a daily protein intake of at least 2 g/kg bodyweight, depending upon the sport. This will automatically be allowed for if the amount of protein is related back to the total energy requirement of the sport. However, there is quite sound physiological reasoning to support a protein intake of at least twice the recommended average.

Research work indicates that protein-rich foods have a stimulatory effect upon the nervous system. They improve the levels of excitation and the associated reflexes. It therefore follows that any sports requiring these qualities, as do sprinting, jumping, tennis, boxing, etc., will benefit in this respect from a higher protein intake. However, it does not follow that any sport not requiring quick reflex actions, such as endurance-based events, has not the same demand for an increase in protein. In fact, this is far from the truth, but for a different reason. During prolonged work, the tissues are affected by 'wear' in much the same way as any machine would be. This wear is in fact a breakdown of all protein, which requires protein for its repair. Thus the nitrogen balance of the body is affected, which necessitates a speedy return to normal; this can only be effected by the protein assimilated from the diet.

Proteins can be divided into first- and second-class varieties which correspond to the number and type of amino-acids present in the protein. The classification also relates to the protein source, whether or not it is of organic or vegetable derivation. Generally speaking, vegetable proteins are inferior to animal proteins. However, there is a trap into which many sportspeople could fall by including only first-class protein in their diet. Certain inferior proteins of the gelatin group yield to the body a substance from which it manufactures creatine. Creatine, when combined with phosphoric acid, produces a substance known as phosphocreatine (CP). See p. 25.

From Chapter 2 it should be remembered that energy is stored in the body in the form of adenosine triphosphate (ATP). Once the store is depleted it is replenished by adding a phosphate bond, from phosphocreatine, to the by-product of the first energy cycle, adenosine diphosphate (ADP). Therefore, gelatin, as a protein, is of value to any person involved in high quality, short duration activities, such as sprinting or jumping.

If insufficient proteins are taken in, the body starts on a katabolic process, by which the cells of the body start to break down and the end result is death. Excessive animal proteins can be harmful as they place an extra strain on the digestive system and can produce toxins on their transit through the digestive tract. Generally speaking, proteins are the most expensive nutrients; those which the body cannot absorb are excreted, so it is poor economy to overload a system merely to produce expensive waste products.

The time of ingestion of protein is also very important. If strength-promoting work such as weight training is to be undertaken, protein should be included in the meal about two hours before the activity. This will mean that the stimulus (weight training) and the raw materials (amino-acids) for strength promotion are available at the same time. Protein should also be included in the final meal of the day (dinner) so that the repair of broken tissue can take place during the night or the period of rest.

If meat, fish, cheese, eggs and fresh vegetables are included in the diet, provided the amount is correct the body should not become deficient in protein. The amount, of course, depends upon the bodyweight of the person and the sport practised. For example, a person involved in the sport of track and field athletics has a requirement of about 25.0 g/kg of meat or meat products per day, and the same amount of milk.

Fats

Very little is said about fats in texts on nutrition. This is probably influenced by the vogue for avoiding animal fats because of their effect upon the production of cholesterol which, it is thought, is contributory to certain heart complaints. However, fats are essential in the diet and form the main provider of energy. The average man has a fat store equal to about 15 per cent of the bodyweight. This represents a massive potential energy system. Earlier in the text (p.39) it was indicated that the potential energy yield of fat is about twice that of carbohydrates or proteins. But fat is not such a good thing as might be suggested because of the relative absence of oxygen from the molecules forming it. It is, therefore, more extravagant in its use of oxygen when metabolised and oxygen is at something of a premium during physical exertion.

Fats are stored in the body as adipose tissue composed of free fatty acids (FFA). With the onset of exercise the adrenal medulla is stimulated to secrete adrenalin (epinephrine), which not only increases the heart rate and blood pressure, but also mobilises FFA for energy production.

Part of this group is the steroid chain which includes the much publicised synthetic male sex hormone used for both its androgenic and anabolic effects. Indeed, it is my opinion that the anabolic steroid has had a most profound effect upon performance levels in most of the power-based sports. This will be covered more fully in chapter 9.

Also included in the group is a substance known as lecethin. Lecethin is a phospholipid and is found in cell membranes, in particular those composing nervous tissue. In this respect, it is thought to act as an insulator surrounding nervous tissue, with the associated hypothesis that it could aid the speed of stimulation to muscles, etc. If the hypothesis is correct, then its presence in the sportsman or woman is essential and the diet should contain lecethin. However, the chances of the body being deficient in lecethin are remote if the recommended amount of organic protein is taken.

In the average man fats account for about 20 per cent of the energy requirements. For those involved in very high work-loads the value increases above this level and for those involved in efforts demanding in excess of 4,000 Calories a day the value approaches 50 per cent.

Fats can be in both animal and vegetable forms. Normally the body must take in its fat requirements as organic fats. However, this does not mean that vegetable fats should be completely excluded from the diet. This is particularly so for people involved in sustained endurance events, where a good deal of energy has to come from the metabolism of fats. The vegetable fats contain a fatty acid which is essential in this situation for the efficient metabolism of fat stores.

The assimilation of fats depends upon their melting point. The higher this is, the more difficult is the fat to assimilate. For example, butter is low on the melting-point scale, so about 97.5 per cent of it is assimilated; other forms are less efficient, with about 90 per cent of vegetable oils being assimilated.

Carbohydrates

Carbohydrates form nature's most efficient source of energy. But, unlike fats, they cannot be stored easily in the body. While it is true to say that the muscles have a small store in the form of muscle glycogen and the liver has a further and much larger store, in the form of liver glycogen, any excess carbohydrates are converted to fats and stored as adipose tissue. However, when carbohydrates are metabolised they are more efficient in their consumption of oxygen during the breakdown process. This is a critical factor for sport because the increased level of activity also makes extra demands upon the oxygen-providing system.

In simple terms carbohydrates exist in two forms – starches and sugars. The sportsman and woman require both but in a controllable ratio. Yakovlev, in an article published by *Physical Culture and Sport* (Moscow 1961) suggests that the ratio should be 64 per cent starches to 36 per cent simple sugars. This supports the commonly held view that sugars act as an irritant to the digestive, nervous and endocrine systems. The sportsperson involved in endurance sports, or ones requiring a high degree of skill and thus the absolute control of this aspect of the nervous system, and who is frequently in a position requiring a carefully controlled secretion of hormones, cannot afford for this aspect of homeostasis to be upset. The recommendation of Yakovlev is supported by most other research workers in the field.

Too great an ingestion of sugars in a short space of time could stimulate the insulin reaction. Insulin is the hormone secreted by a group of specialised cells forming part of the pancreas and its function is to control the critical balance of blood sugars. On the other hand, starches are absorbed gradually into the system, in harmony with their rate of digestion, and do not cause a rapid increase in blood sugar levels.

Carbohydrates are easily provided for in the diet, as most of the common foods are high in this nutrient. For example, bread and cereals contain 50–70 per cent carbohydrates, and potatoes about 15 per cent. Honey is an easily assimilated carbohydrate, but is part of the sugar group and should be taken as part of the 36 per cent of sugars included in the diet. Even in countries where the level of nutrition is poor, where, for example, the staple diet is rice or millet, the people will never be short of carbohydrates.

Vitamins

Up to this point in the text, the general theme regarding nutrients has been one of supply and demand, associated with energy requirements. As far as energy is concerned, it is a fairly accurate generalisation to suggest that if more of everything is eaten the energy requirements will be met. However, this is certainly not so as far as vitamins are concerned. With only a modicum of knowledge of nutritional science it is easy to identify the foods rich in the basic nutrients, but to recognise those foods which can supply the body's requirements of vitamins demands a much deeper study. Hence, the simple idea of supply and demand takes on a new meaning, because it is difficult to assess the demand, and not an easy task to identify the supply. One thing is certain; the research work emanating from nations whose prowess in sport is instantly recognisable, suggests that vitamin therapy is essential for those involved in high-level sport. Unfortunately, the medical fraternity, by and large, remains unconvinced. Specialists in sports nutrition are adamant that the more intense the metabolism, the greater is the body's need for vitamins.

Research work in Russia, Finland and East Germany, prompted by the nation's desire to be successful in sport, established that the addition of the vitamin B group and vitamin C enhanced the effectiveness of training. The resulting hypothesis was that these vitamins aided the training function by increasing the body's capacity for work, reducing the fatigue factor and hastening the recovery process. It is possible to support these conclusions bio-chemically.

The general opinion of those doctors associated with national sports medicine is that there is little evidence to support the need for vitamin therapy. They stand firm in their belief that the average British diet provides all of the nutrients and vitamins in quantities to satisfy the needs of even the most active sportsman. However, the recommendations of sports scientists from both Russia and Finland seem to have the backing of valid research.

Yakovlev, in *Physical Culture and Sport* (Moscow 1961), recommends the following for athletes during various phases of their training.

Table 5 *Recommended vitamin intakes for athletes during different phases of training*

Training period	Explosive events						Endurance events					
	A mg	B_1 mg	B_2 mg	Ncn mg	C mg	E mg	A mg	B_1 mg	B_2 mg	Ncn mg	C mg	E mg
active recovery	2	2.5	2	20	75	3	2	3	2	20	100	3
period of principal training	3	5	2.5	20	150	3	3	10	5	25	250	6
competition period	2	10	5	25	150	3	2	15	5	25	300	

Seppo Nuuttila, Director of Coaching in Finland, in a paper presented to a symposium for sportsmen and women in London in November 1973, suggested that dieticians studying sports nutrition in Finland recommended the following intake of vitamins during periods of intensive endurance training:

A	B_1	B_2	Ncn	C	E
3.3 mg	2.5-5 mg	2.6-5 mg	20 mg	100-250 mg	30-60 mg

Apart from the increase in vitamin E, the Russian and Finnish figures almost directly correspond with each other.

For comparison, the following table lists the daily recommended intake of nutrients for 18-35–year–olds in the UK.

Table 6 *Recommended daily intake of nutrients for 18-35–year–olds*

Occupation	Energy require-ment Cal	Protein g	B$_1$ mg	B$_2$ mg	Niacin mg	C	A micro g	D micro g	Calcium mg	Iron mg
Sedentary	2,700	68	1.1	1.7	18	30	750	2.5	500	10
Moderately active	3,000	75	1.2	1.7	18	30	750	2.5	500	10
Very active	3,600	90	1.4	1.7	18	30	750	2.5	500	10

An interesting point arising from this table is that in terms of top-level sport 3,600 Cal is not very high and some sportsmen double this figure in their training. The levels of all the vitamins, particularly vitamin C, are well down on those recommended by the Russian and Finnish surveys.

The Canadian dietary standards for the vitamin B group are as follows:

Table 7 *Canadian dietary standards for the vitamin B group*

energy requirement Cal	B$_1$ mg	B$_2$ mg	niacin mg
2,850	0.9	1.4	9
4,900	1.5	2.5	15

The following is an extract from a report by the Warsaw Nutrition Laboratory with reference to their Olympic team: 'The long-distance runner may use up to 6,400 Cal per day but when left to his own devices tends to consume extra Calories as fats and carbohydrates and becomes deficient in Vitamin C.'

While the precise role of vitamins is not fully understood, it is certain that their action is that of a catalyst aiding a chemical reaction, or reactions, which might involve other catalysts. Hence, at times, they produce a chain-like reaction with a large degree of interdependence. Several papers on nutrition, with research back-up, suggest that athletes involved in heavy training loads, particularly in endurance situations, require additional amounts of vitamin B_6 in the region of 3–6 mg per day. Vitamin B_6 increases the body's need for vitamin B_1 so this must be allowed for if that type of therapy is considered necessary.

Certain vitamins, particularly B_1, B_{12} and E, have a stimulatory effect, so it would be unwise to take them in the late evening for fear of disrupting sleep. Without this sort of information it would be very easy to lose on the roundabouts what you are gaining on the swings.

At present, many people throughout the world who are involved in sports science and nutrition appear to be focusing a lot of attention on vitamin B_{12} and vitamin B_{14} (pangamic acid). The understanding is that they have a considerable effect upon the production of energy at muscle cell level. Valid research to support this hypothesis seems hard to come by; evidence of top-class sportsmen and women having fairly frequent injections of vitamin B_{12} and vitamin B_{14} through biopangamine is readily available. While such injections might be easy to dismiss as having merely a psychological effect, their use among athletes from very sophisticated sporting nations might suggest that the latter have evidence supporting the use of B_{12} and B_{14} as an enzyme in the production of energy.

From the facts so far, it would seem that the world of vitamins is a confused one, with even the world's experts failing to agree on precise figures. It must be remembered that one is dealing with tiny amounts and where the research work indicates a large discrepancy between different conclusions, it could be associated with the understanding, or lack of it, concerning work loads and energy requirements. It is not my intention in this chapter to put forward a personal opinion. This will follow later. My intention is to put forward what appears to be valid research work so that readers can arrive at their own conclusion, using the information how they think best.

From the discussion so far in this chapter, the reader might be tempted to form the opinion that only the vitamin B group has any significant effect upon the body as far as sport is concerned. This conclusion would be incorrect, but as the B group is a very large and important one, it is natural that it should become a focal point.

The sportsman and woman involved in very high training loads are constantly breaking down muscle protein, which has to be re-established in conjunction with the growth hormone and protein which is part of the dietary intake. Irrespective of any form of protein therapy, the sportsperson should naturally take in more protein than the average individual. It is generally recognised that there is a very close relationship between protein and vitamin A. In fact, research workers, particularly those from the Hebrew University in Rehovot, now know that if protein is fed to undernourished and malnourished people it can do more harm than good. However, if it is given in conjunction with vitamin A then a therapeutic effect takes place. Other workers in the field have observed that vitamin A deficiency occurs simultaneously with protein malnutrition and that increased protein intake demands a greater intake of vitamin A.

Vitamin A is a fat-soluble vitamin which participates in a number of biochemical processes. The first and most important one is concerned with its association with protein and growth. However, it is also known to have an effect upon vision, particularly in failing and artificial light. Some sports have always been subject to artificial light, and the list is growing – now we are hearing of cricket matches played under floodlighting. Other sports rely heavily upon this form of lighting to extend training and practice time. To get the full benefit, it would appear that vitamin A is essential.

While people who have a high intake of vegetables and dairy products are unlikely to be low in this vitamin, those who have tried to eliminate cholesterol from their diet by avoiding eggs, dairy products, etc. could be in danger of the level falling too low, and vitamin A therapy might just tip the scales. It must be remembered, though, that vitamin A is a fat-soluble vitamin and that an excess could become toxic. However, most of the athletes I know take an excess of dairy products and will be unlikely to become low in this vitamin. If supplementation is thought necessary a daily dose of fish oil will certainly be a cheap insurance policy.

Vitamin C is the vitamin with which the majority of people are familiar, and many are only too eager to associate most of the common ailments, ranging from spots to colds, with its deficiency.

To a large extent their belief is correct, for most authorities recognise vitamin C as a virus killer. The top-class sportsman and woman cannot afford to have competition or training either restricted or terminated because of minor infection; contrary to widespread belief, training does not ensure against virus infections and if the truth were known the athlete might be more susceptible to this type of infection than the ordinary person. Following the belief that prevention is better than cure, and bearing in mind that the two countries listed earlier advocate a high intake of vitamin C, it would appear that there are perfectly valid reasons for attempting to increase one's intake of this vitamin.

There is an association between vitamin C and iron therapy, which is well recognised by all branches of the medical profession. As it is the iron pigment in the haemoglobin which carries the oxygen, the vital fuel for muscular work, the sportsman and woman cannot afford to be short of this simple vitamin. However, its effect will be more fully discussed under the section on iron and iron therapy.

To take the discussion of vitamin C a stage further, Dr. Linus Pauling of the USA, at the second International Conference of Social Psychiatry in London in 1969, suggested that vitamin C has a profound effect upon mental health. Researchers have found that there is a higher concentration of vitamin C in the brain and associated tissue than in any other tissue in the body. The findings probably support the fact that the brain requires vitamin C. The sportsman or woman certainly needs to be alert and to have the degree of neuromuscular control essential for the execution of the intricate skills involved in most sports.

Vitamin preparations are constantly subject to commercial exploitation and the one which must surely head the list is vitamin E. This is certainly because of its possible effect upon libido, which has helped to give it the name of the 'sex vitamin'. Research workers have studied its effect upon a wide number of diseases, mainly associated with circulatory defects at all levels. This area of research has prompted the supporters of vitamin E to suggest that its effect is at tissue level, reducing the demand for oxygen. It has also been suggested that it aids the dispersal of fresh blood clots and dilates blood vessels, with an associated limitation of scar tissue. Both of these findings could have a profound effect upon sport.

All of the endurance-based sports are looking for economy in the use of oxygen at tissue level. This could be a factor that could control the delicate balance of true success or failure, and as such cannot be ignored. All sportsmen and women, at some time, suffer injury where the formation of scar tissue could restrict their return to active participation. Indeed, in many cases success or failure in a sport can be attributed to the speed of rehabilitation after injury. Many good sportsmen and women have been forced into premature retirement due to the frustration associated with a prolonged absence from training forced by injury. Anything that could possibly help to avoid this situation would obviously benefit sport.

The magazine *Prevention* of December 1971 lists a research article from the *American Journal of Clinical Nutrition* by Drs Leonard and Losowsky, St James's Hospital, Leeds, linking the life of red blood cells with vitamin E. As the red blood cells are the oxygen transporters, the effect of this finding upon sport should be instantly recognisable.

A very recent addition to the library of nutrition is one by Dr Damien Downing, *Day light robbery*. Dr Downing practises nutritional medicine in York and is a founder of the British Society for nutritional medicine. In the test he highlights the need for sunlight and the effect that this has upon vitamin D and C and of the danger of continually working all day under narrow spectrum artificial light. Furthermore, it is impossible to compensate for this by using the normal 'sun beds', as again these only work on a very narrow band from the sunlight spectrum. Research indicates that 'widespectrum' lighting can have the same effect as sunlight, bringing with it all of the advantages of its rays. Other than the cosmetic effect of a sun tan, in particular it helps increase levels of testosterone, the essential hormone in strength building.

Minerals

Mineral balance is as important to the sportsman and woman as vitamin presence. A brief survey of the possible effect of minerals upon the total health of an individual is therefore essential for a text of this nature.

Yakovlev, in *Physical Culture and Sport* (Moscow 1961), a translation appearing in *Track Technique* No. 23 (March 1966), suggests that the athlete in training must have a proportional increase in minerals. The following table compares the daily requirements for the average person with Yakovlev's suggestion for the sportsman and woman.

	calcium	iron	magnesia	phosphor	sodium chloride
average person	0.8	15 mg	0.5 g	1.25 g	20 g
active sportsman	1.0-1.75 g	20 mg	0.8 g	1.5-2.5 g	25-30 g

It is difficult to find valid research supporting the needs of increased mineral intake. However, an additional survey to that given in Chapter 2, illustrating the functions of minerals, might help to give empirical support.

Calcium While calcium is readily linked with an efficient bone structure, essential for all contact sports, it is said to have an effect upon cardiac rhythm and neuro-muscular excitation, both of which must be at peak efficiency for high-level sport participation.

Phosphor has a similar role in assuring the correct functioning of the neuro-muscular system. It also has an association with the functioning of certain vitamins and with sugar metabolism, a good source of energy.

Iron is quickly recognised as an essential mineral for sportsmen and women, particularly those involved in endurance events. However, this again is an area where those involved with sports medicine have opinions differing from those in general practice. The difference certainly arises from what is considered satisfactory for the average person in comparison with those involved in high training loads. There are also several different methods for indicating the various levels relating to iron, which tends to confuse the layman.

Iron is the essential pigment for the formation of haemoglobin, the oxygen transporter. Without iron it is estimated that the human body would need over 300 litres (approx 530 pints) of bloods to transport its oxygen requirements; with it the amount drops to about 5 litres (8 pints). The extra weight involved in carrying this amount of fluid would certainly not aid man in his mobility.

Because it is the haemoglobin that carries over 99 per cent of the body's oxygen, the haemoglobin content of the blood is most important. The average blood count for men is 14.7 g/100 cc of blood and for women 13.7 g/100 cc. If the level falls below 12g/100 cc, the condition is known as anaemia. However, these levels bear little resemblance to the figures one would expect from a very fit middle distance runner. In this respect one is looking for a blood count of at least 100 (per cent) or 15.8 g/100 cc in men and at least 95 (per cent) or 13.7/100 cc in women.

It must be remembered that women can lose up to 70 ml (2.5 fl oz) of blood during the menstrual period, which represents quite a considerable loss of iron. Hence, women are more likely to be anaemic and in need of iron therapy.

As a coach I have learned to spot the possible symptoms of iron deficiency in athletes. They include general observations of pallor, sudden deterioration in training or racing performances, breathlessness and complaints of headaches and insomnia. Any combination of these factors now prompts me to recommend a visit to the doctor for a blood test and for the doctor to take the appropriate action. In some cases this has necessitated an injection or therapy using iron preparations together with vitamin C. The indiscriminate use of iron therapy should be condemned; it can prove toxic to the liver and can affect the viscosity of the blood, which in turn affects its ease of transportation.

While there are other minerals, such as zinc, copper and magnesia, which have a close interaction with the vitamins, as was discussed in Chapter 1, there only remains sodium chloride, or common salt, to discuss. In sport, particularly events such as marathon races, and especially when events are held in humid countries, there is ample evidence of the side-effects of fluid and salt loss. Almost any disturbance of the salt balance of the body will affect performance, the amount to which it is affected being almost directly proportional to the disturbance. For example, a minor disturbance might only manifest itself in a degree of lassitude, but at the other end of the scale are heat cramp and prostration.

In concluding this section, I would like to highlight some very recent research which is being conducted in American schools and prisons, and is supported by some work in British schools. Both are ongoing. The researchers have suggested that a lack of certain nutrients and vitamins/minerals impairs intellectual capacity, affects performance in examinations and contributes to certain forms of anti-social behaviour. Furthermore, the situations respond to nutritional therapy.

6

Food supplements and vitamin therapy

Certainly one of the most controversial topics in sports nutrition must be whether or not food supplements or vitamin therapy are necessary. The basic answer, for most people, is a very simple and logical one. If the sportsman or woman eats well, from a good mixed diet of natural foods, there will be no need to supplement the diet at all. Unfortunately, in this era of mass-produced food, freezing, canning, preserving and storing, the nutritional value of many foods is reduced.

Sport at the top level is almost essentially for the young, a group of people who often come from student populations and have to rely upon mass catering, which is the poorest method for producing meals and at the same time retaining the full nutritive values of the original food. Similarly, there are tremendous demands upon the leisure time of this group. As well as satisfying the demands of their sport, most have social commitments, the total effect of which is to make time a premium. After a day of work or study there is often no time to relax over a well-prepared meal and allow the necessary time for it to digest. Hence, time is invariably reclaimed at the expense of meals. Many young sportsmen and women rush direct from their place of employment to their training venue and expect to get the full training value from an empty tank. In this situation most eat well after they have completed their training programme, at a time when sleep and intestinal activity should be the main priority.

With just this brief glimpse into the daily life of most sports-people, it can be seen that their life-style is not that of the average person and so their dietary needs are different. Admittedly, some appreciate the need to devote as much care and thought to their nutritional needs as they do to their training programmes, and allow for this in their daily programme. Invariably, these sportsmen and women live at home and receive the benefit of devoted parents singularly committed to the achievement of sporting excellence.

Training time

One of the main problems facing sportsmen and women is the training time relative to the ingestion of food. For those who have to fit in their training after a day's work, the problem is even more complex. Most sportsmen and women commence their training during the week at about 7 p.m. It is preferable to allow a digestive period of about two hours between a meal and the commencement of training. This would almost certainly make the best meal-time coincide with the final period at work, or the period spent commuting between work and home. On the surface there appear to be three possible compromises:

1. To eat at the normal lunch-break period of about 1 p.m. and not eat again until after training. This will create the 'empty tank' syndrome.

2. To rush a meal after work and risk the discomfort of training on a full stomach.

3. To eat at lunch-time and take a snack during the commuting period.

The last solution is, in my opinion, the wisest of the compromises, especially if a quickly digested food supplement (or in some cases a meal substitute) is used. A number of manufacturing companies specialise in this type of food, their primary concern being to cater for the needs of hospital patients requiring special nutritional therapy. Brand names which have appeared include Nutriment and Ensure, both from an American source. Invariably the 'food' is canned and in the form of a drink. These preparations can add considerably to the daily food budget as they are expensive when used as supplements, but the ingestion of a glucose drink, glucose candy bar or a quick sandwich snack is almost certainly the greater of two evils.

It is my personal opinion that such a situation should be avoided, as I can never see it producing excellence. It might be suggested that the alternative to this is the full-time sportsman or woman who is free to train at the most convenient time of the day. I am convinced that we are fast approaching this situation, or a situation where the top sportspeople are released from their employment at a convenient time, most conducive to a proper training effect.

Nutritional therapy

It is most unlikely that any athlete following the most severe training programme will require any form of fat or carbohydrate therapy. Of the three main nutritional categories, this leaves only protein therapy.

Like most aspects of nutritional science, the suggestion of protein therapy is a controversial issue. Both schools of thought, for and against, have their supporters and their critics. It is my personal opinion that any sportsman or woman placed in the situation where he or she has to rely upon mass-produced foods and quick snacks requires some form of protein therapy. While the health food manufacturers come under a great deal of criticism from the medical profession, they do appear to cater for this market. The sportsman or woman placed in this situation should make him or herself familiar with what is available on the market and then make a choice. However, I must emphasise that it is a compromise, and also raises the issue of natural versus synthetic foods, which will be discussed later in the text.

A parallel issue is the possible psychological effect that could be brought about by nutritional therapy. Sportspeople often convince themselves that they have a nutritional deficiency and will not be swayed by the opinions of a doctor, adviser or coach. In this situation I would certainly condone most forms of nutritional therapy, especially that of protein. There is quite sound evidence to support the conclusion that excess protein is harmless and that it is merely converted to another usable product and metabolised in the normal way.

While it would appear difficult to justify any supplementation of fats or carbohydrates, other than those involved with specialised diets such as the 'Saltin', the supplementation of amino acids might be worth consideration. Indeed, the whole area of free form amino acid supplementation is the vogue conversation point among those interested in sports' nutrition. The issue has probably been accelerated by the fear of detection when using other ergogenic aids, which has sparked off the interest in other forms of legal therapy. High on the priority list for consideration is the supplementation of amino acids such as argenine and ornithine. These are said to have an effect upon muscle growth through the action of the growth hormone and upon the secretion of insulin and glucagon, both of which have an effect upon the availability of energy. However, the field of study is a fairly recent one and as yet there is little valid supporting evidence.

As far as vitamin therapy is concerned, I agree with the ideas put forward by Yakovlev and Nuuttila which were outlined in Chapter 5. I am convinced that even for sportsmen and women, who enjoy a well-balanced, mixed diet, and who are involved in very heavy training loads, a degree of vitamin therapy is essential. Here it is wise to use the relatively inexpensive supplements readily available, without prescription, from most chemists or health food shops. These include wheat-germ oil, brewer's yeast and ascorbic acid, which will provide all of the vitamin B and C a sportsperson is likely to require. A personal favourite, but slightly more expensive, is one of the pollen extracts such as Pollitabs or Pollenaps. Research work based in Sweden, Italy, Poland and France and presented at the International Symposium on Nutrition for Sportsmen at Crystal Palace, London, in November 1973, all showed that pollenic extracts had a marked effect upon improved performances, compared with control groups, in several sports including weight-lifting, Association football and athletics. The findings here also supported those presented to a similar symposium in Helsingborg, Sweden in July 1972. This symposium included a paper by J. Dubnisay (Paris) on a clinical trial of a pollenic extract with patients suffering from anorexia (loss of appetite). The results indicated a very positive response, similar to that which is produced by artificial anabolic hormones. I have also used pollenic extracts in several areas of sport and found them to be most beneficial. There is also an associated euphoric effect which would be difficult to condemn as a mere placebo advantage.

Analysis showed that cernitin pollen extract contained several essential amino-acids, vitamins, magnesia, iron, cobalt, copper, zinc and manganese. In other words, it could be an excellent multi-vitamin for those who wish to take out that little extra insurance policy. I must emphasise that, like any other form of vitamin therapy, it should be used as a supplement to a good diet and not as a prop to support a poor one. I am a firm believer that the 'natural source' is best and that the nutritional elements should be taken by eating the right things. This will be further discussed in Chapter 7.

Iron therapy is one area where those involved with the study of sports medicine reach some degree of harmony with athletes. I believe that periodic iron therapy, particularly with women and those involved in sustained endurance events, can enhance performance.

Ideally, any form of iron therapy should be given by a doctor following a blood count. However, this is not always possible and in some nations it is influenced by the direction of a national health scheme. Most people in sports medicine seem to prescribe Ferrograd 'C', which is a fairly expensive preparation. The same effect can be obtained by combining Fersamal with ascorbic acid. Fersamal tablets contain 65 mg of iron fumerate, a soluble version of iron with few side-effects. The daily dose should be two or three tablets taken with two tablets of 50 mg of ascorbic acid. A possible side-effect might be mild constipation, which could be corrected with a bran breakfast cereal.

This type of vitamin/mineral therapy comes within the self-administered category, and is open to any sportsman or woman who shares my opinion that food supplements represent an avenue that could lead to greater success, and as such must be explored. However, I am also of the opinion that vitamin B_{12} injections can enhance the performance of those involved in explosive events. This type of therapy does not come into the above category and must only be administered by the team doctor.

In concluding this chapter I would like to emphasise that sport makes heavy demands upon the financial resources of the performer and that money spent indiscriminately on food supplements might be better directed elsewhere.

7

Planning a diet for sportsmen and women

It is not the intention of this chapter to give a typical breakfast, lunch and dinner menu for the sportsman or woman to follow. This would be impossible as there are so many foods from which to select, with almost as many personal likes and dislikes. Rather, it is my intention to provide a number of tables listing the foods commonly eaten, together with their nutritional composition.

When interpreting table 8 it must be remembered that certain foods are enriched with vitamins or protein. The vitamin value of certain foods varies with the time of year and with storage. Except where stated, the value refers to the uncooked food; with cooking the nutritional value of food changes. The table is taken from the Manual of Nutrition, Ministry of Agriculture and Fisheries, published by HMSO.

The table illustrates that there is no such thing as the complete food, though probably the nearest to it is milk. In the main, the foods which I have selected are those most commonly used in the British diet. It can be observed that certain foods such as meat, fish, bread and eggs contain a greater range of nutrients than sugars and preserves, etc. Hence it is wise planning to include more of the first group of foods in the diet.

With reference to the table, it is most important to make clear the distinction between nutrient content of food and nutrient contribution in diet. For example, the nutrient content of peas in very high when compared with that of potatoes, but because a far greater weight of potatoes than peas is consumed, the contribution of peas is less. In the field of minerals, potatoes contain only 0.5-0.7 mg/100 g of iron, which is low when compared with liver, which is relatively rich in iron at 11.4-15.0 mg/100 g. Although the iron content of liver is some twenty times higher than that of potatoes, liver only contributes about 4 per cent of the iron in the average diet, whereas potatoes contribute about 7 per cent. Table 9 will give a wider understanding of the contribution certain foods make to our average diet.

Table 8 *Composition of foods per 100g*

Food	Protein g	Fat g	Carbo-hydrate g	Water g	Calcium mg	Iron mg	Vitamins					
							A micro g	B₁ mg	B₂ mg	B₃ mg	C mg	D micro g
beef	18.1	17.1		64	7	1.9	0	0.06	0.19	8.1	0	0
lamb	15.9	30.2		53	7	1.3	0	0.09	0.19	7.4	0	0
pork	15.8	29.6		54	8	0.8	0	0.58	0.16	6.9	0	0
chicken	20.8	6.7		73	11	1.5	0	0.04	0.17	9.5	0	0
liver	20.7	8.0	2.2	69	6	11.4	6,000	0.26	3.10	18.1	30	0.75
bacon	14.4	40.5	0	41	7	1.0	0	0.36	0.14	5.8	0	0
sausages (beef)	9.6	24.1	11.7	50	48	1.4	0	0.03	0.13	7.1	0	0
fish	17.4	0.7	0	82	16	0.3	0	0.08	0.07	4.8	0	0
eggs	12.3	10.9	0	75	54	2.1	140	0.09	0.47	3.7	0	1.5
milk	3.3	3.8	4.8	88	120	0.1	44	0.04	0.15	0.9	1	0.05
cheese	25.4	34.5	0	37	810	0.6	420	0.04	0.50	5.2	0	0.35
butter	0.5	81.0	0	16	15	0.2	995	0	0	0.1	0	1.25
margarine	0.2	81.5	0	15	4	0.3	900	0	0	0.1	0	8.00
jam	0.5	0	69.2	30	18	12.0	2	0	0	0	0	0
honey	0.4	0	76.4	23	50	0.4	0	0	0	0.2	10	0
beans (runner)	2.2	0	3.9	89	27	0.8	50	0.05	0.05	1.4	20	0
cabbage	2.8	0	2.8	88	57	0.6	50	0.06	0.10	0.7	53	0
carrots	0.7	0	5.4	90	48	0.6	2,000	0.06	0.05	0.7	6	0
peas	5.8	0	10.6	84	15	1.9	50	0.32	0.15	3.5	25	0
potato chips	3.8	9.0	37.3	48	14	1.4	0	0.10	0.15	2.2	6	0
potatoes (boiled)	1.4	0	19.7	81	4	0.5	5	0.08	0.04	1.2	6	0
apples	0.3	0	12.0	84	4	0.3	0	0.04	0.03	0.1	5	0
bananas	1.1	0	19.2	71	7	0.4	33	0.04	0.02	0.8	10	0
oranges	0.8	0	8.5	86	41	0.3	8	0.10	0.07	0.3	50	0
nuts (almonds)	20.5	53.5	4.3	5	247	4.2	0	0.32	0.25	4.9	0	0
bread (white)	8.0	1.7	54.3	39	100	1.7	0	0.18	0.03	2.6	0	0
bread (brown)	9.2	1.4	48.3	39	88	2.5	0	0.28	0.07	2.7	0	0
cornflakes	7.4	0.4	85.4	2	5	0.3	0	1.13	1.41	10.6	0	0
rice	6.2	1.0	86.8	12	4	0.4	0	0.08	0.03	1.5	0	0
instant coffee	4.0	0.7	35.5	2	140	4.0	0	0	0.10	45.7	0	0
tea	0	0	0	0	0	0	0	0	0	0.9	6	0

When the average British diet is considered, it is convenient to divide the wide variety of foodstuffs consumed into six basic categories, as illustrated in tables 9a and b. It is true that not all items of our diet are included in this grouping, but anything outside the grouping will make only a very small contribution to our total nutritional requirements.

Table 9a *Percentage contribution made by important foods in the average diet*

food group	calories	protein	fat	calcium	iron
milk, cheese, eggs	15	29	21	63	6
meat/fish	16	31	30	4	29
cereals (bread, etc.)	31	29	11	22	33
fruit/vegetables	10	10	1	8	22
fats (butter, etc.)	15	1	36	1	—
sugars/preserves	12	—	—	—	—

Table 9b *Percentage contribution made by important foods in the average diet*

food group	vitamins					
	A	B_1	B_2	B_3	C	D
milk, cheese, eggs	23	17	51	4	9	26
meat/fish	22	25	21	40	1	26
cereals (bread, etc.)	2	32	7	28	1	3
fruit/vegetables	27	25	13	21	87	—
fats (butter, etc.)	26	1	1	1	—	43
sugars/preserves	—	—	1	1	1	—

From tables 9a and b we can see the important contribution that certain food groups make to our diet. Dairy products and eggs make a massive contribution, providing at least 10 per cent of our total Calorie requirements, about 20 per cent of our protein and over 50 per cent of our calcium requirements. Meat and fish make a major contribution to our total nutritional needs in all but calcium and vitamin C. Cereals provide most of the carbohydrates required and contribute about 30 per cent of the total energy requirements. They also make a major contribution to our protein and vitamin intake, because most flours are now enriched after the milling process, which tends to reduce the natural quality of the cereal.

Fruit and vegetables are important mainly for their contribution to the total vitamin needs, as illustrated in table 9b.

Tables 8 and 9 provide us with a very simple solution to the nutritional needs of sportsmen and women. If we eat well from each of the six basic groupings, we are certain to include all of the nutritional requirements for an active body. So, the simple cereal plus egg for breakfast, and meat or fish plus vegetables for lunch and dinner, combined with the milk and sweeteners in the associated beverages, are bound to at least direct us along the right road.

All that the sportsman or woman requires to head in the right direction is a well-balanced, nutritionally adequate diet, which can be obtained by following these simple rules.

1. Each meal should contain some foods rich in protein, i.e. meat, poultry, fish, cheese, eggs, milk or bread.
2. Each main meal should contain fruit and vegetables, which are good sources of vitamins and minerals.
3. Energy-rich foods such as fats, bread, cakes, biscuits, and confectionery should be sufficient to satisfy the appetite and to maintain correct bodyweight.

There is one simple trap which the sportsman or woman could fall into; he/she must recognise that the most expensive is not necessarily the best. The British are famed and recognised for their love of fish and chips. Originally this meal was carefully introduced to the public as a cheap, well-balanced meal. Of course the cost of providing fish has now overtaken our society, which no longer makes it a very cheap meal, but its popularity has not diminished. The cheaper cuts of meat, while they might require extra preparation, are just as nutritious as the expensive cuts. The list below gives some of the cheaper foods to cover each of the nutritional categories.

Protein – bread, milk, cheese, potatoes, baked beans, chicken, eggs, breakfast cereal, liver, fish.

Carbohydrates – sugar, bread, potatoes, breakfast cereal.

Calcium – milk, cheese, carrots.

Iron – liver, baked beans, potatoes, bread, peas, fresh green vegetables.

Vitamin A – carrots, liver, margarine, butter, cheese, milk.

Vitamin B_1 – fortified breakfast cereal, bread, peas, milk, pork.

Vitamin B_2 – liver, fortified breakfast cereal, milk, eggs, cheese.

Vitamin B_3 – fortified breakfast cereal, potatoes, liver, bread,

chicken.
Vitamin C – fruit juices, oranges, fresh green vegetables, tomatoes, peas.
Vitamin D – margarine, butter, eggs, fatty fish.

The foods are listed in order of cheapness compared with the amount one would need to eat to get the same nutritional benefits.

The nutritional importance of a food depends upon the following factors.
1. The composition of the raw food – allowances must be made for inedible waste.
2. The amount of the particular foodstuff eaten.
3. The extent to which nutrients are lost during preparation, cooking, storing, seasonal changes, etc.

Allowances have to be made in tables 8 and 9 and the list above for the first two of these points. Reference has also been made to these topics earlier in this chapter. It only remains to discuss the effect of preparation, cooking and preserving on the foods.

Most foods have to be prepared and cooked before they can be eaten. For some foods, such as fresh fruit and vegetables when eaten raw, the journey from original state to the table is a very simple one. For others it is much more complicated, as in the production of flour, where the inedible parts have to be removed during milling and the flour subsequently prepared and baked before it reaches us in edible form. At each stage of the process, some of the nutrients are discarded or destroyed.

Cooking
Heat causes chemical and physical changes in food which generally make the food more palatable or digestible. However, generally speaking cooking reduces the nutritional value of food. This reduction can be minimised if, for example, the water in which vegetables are cooked is used in the preparation of gravies, etc., and the fat in which meat is cooked used in soups or for recooking other meats, etc.

Freezing
This method of preserving reduces the vitamin content, especially with vegetables, and particularly vitamin C. However, it represents the most economical method, as far as keeping the nutritional value of the original food is concerned, when compared with the other methods of preserving.

Heat processing
Canning and bottling reduces the value of the heat-sensitive vitamins

of the of the B and C groups particularly. The loss depends upon the level of heat required and the duration of its application in the preserving process.

Storage of fresh food, particularly in some cases in daylight, will reduce the nutritive value of the food. The simple answer to this is to try to eat the food as fresh as possible.

In basic terms, heating reduces the protein, mineral and vitamin A, B, and C content of foods. Storage in light and air reduces the vitamin content of most foods. The addition of an acid or alkali also reduces the vitamin content.

Vitamin C is probably the least stable of all vitamins. It is partially destroyed in water, and very readily destroyed by air. Vitamin D is stable in most normal cooking procedures, as is vitamin E. Vitamin E, however, is less stable when released to air.

At this stage, it might be worthwhile to select certain items of common foodstuffs and discuss the effect of cooking, preserving, etc., on their nutritional content.

Milk When milk is heated the protein content forms a skin on the top of the milk, so the skin should not be discarded.

To preserve milk, it is subjected to various kinds of heat treatment. In this case, the fat-soluble vitamins are relatively unchanged but the protein value is affected. Sterilising, which is a much harsher form of heat treatment, considerably reduces the vitamin B and C content. In skimmed milk, the fat and fat-soluble vitamins are removed but most of the protein and calcium content are retained.

Eggs When eggs are cooked there is a slight reduction in the protein content and some of the B vitamins are lost. However, generally speaking eggs respond well to several forms of cooking.

Meat When meat is cooked it shrinks and a proportion of its nutritional value passes into the 'drip' or is dissolved in the cooking water. However, after cooking the levels of vitamin B and A are not drastically reduced.

Fish The cooking of fish produces a similar effect to that given for meat. The protein value is slightly reduced and a certain amount of the water-soluble vitamins disappear into the stock, but the fat-soluble vitamins remain almost unchanged.

Vegetables The main purpose of cooking vegetables is to soften the cellular tissue. Between 50 and 70 per cent of the vitamin C content of fruit and vegetables is lost during cooking. With potatoes, this loss can be reduced if the potato is cooked in the jacket.

Cereals Most flour is now vitamin-enriched. However, when it is converted to bread, pastry, etc. a certain amount of the vitamins are lost.

The sportsman or woman will certainly require three main meals each day and will probably need to space them with a snack. However, snacks can have the effect of reducing one's appetite for the subsequent main meal. This is particularly the case when too much sweet stuff is eaten at the snack. Breakfast is a relatively important meal for the athlete. There is very little nutritional difference between a hot and cold breakfast, so in this respect it is a matter of personal choice.

As already outlined, the problem facing the sportsman and woman is not just one of what to eat, but also when to eat it. The top-class sportsperson who has to spend a relatively large amount of his or her time training or competing, cannot make quite the same allowances for eating and digestion times as the normal person. In view of this, any time-saving aid will be beneficial. Foods which will reduce mastication time can help, especially if they are used in conjunction with food supplements. Both soup and alcohol have a speeding-up effect on the digestive process. It might not be just accidental that many meals have a soup course and are frequently accompanied by wine! These are all factors which must be taken into account when planning a menu for a sportsman or woman.

The final consideration must be the type of sport and the duration of the activity. However, this will be influenced by the somatotype (body-type) of the participant. Generally speaking, the different sports attract certain body-types specific to that sport. Also, within the same sport, different positions or events attract different body-types. The classic examples of this are track and field athletics and the versions of rugby football. For example, it is unlikely that one will find a heavy scrum-half, a light prop-forward, a very heavy hockey player or a light discus thrower. Certain physiques are best suited to certain sports and the chances of finding the wrong somatotype for the sport, at the top level, are most unlikely. It is a question of simple mechanics; the heavy person is unsuited to sustained endurance sports and the light person is unsuited to heavy contact sports. If the simple advice given earlier in the text, where the diet is related to bodyweight, is followed, the performer is unlikely to be deficient in any area of nutrition. Basically, the person involved in heavy contact sports, which require a large muscle bulk, will need more protein, and the person involved in sustained endurance events will need more carbohydrates.

There are some sports, such as boxing, wrestling and weight-lifting, that require their competitors to keep within certain weight limits. The answer here must be to pick the category related to one's natural bodyweight and then eat the necessary foods to keep the weight fairly constant. It is unwise to starve or dehydrate to make a lower category, or overeat to move up into a higher category. Both are likely to put the competitor at a disadvantage. In these sports, very careful monitoring of the bodyweight before meals, after meals, after training, etc. is essential, so that it becomes possible to predict what effect each of the variables will have upon the weight of the competitor.

Pre-event meals and very special considerations for the marathon runner or distance skier will be discussed in the next chapter.

8

The pre-event meal and special diets

It is my opinion that this area of sports nutrition is probably the most abused of any we have so far discussed. One still hears of the first division soccer sides that include beefsteak, sherry and eggs, etc. in their pre-match meal. While it might be possible to support this from a psychological point of view, it can only be condemned as unsound nutritional practice. I can also recall talking to a top-class distance runner who happened to have a good race after a meal of steak pie and chips and would not subsequently consider anything else for his pre-event meal.

While it is true to say that most people are unlikely to perform well on a full stomach, it is equally true to say that they will not perform well when the time interval between the competition and their last meal is excessive. So the problem is what to eat and when.

What to eat

Before an event the body requires food that will help to provide enough energy for the duration of the event. It must be remembered that the body has a store of energy and that the pre-event meal performs the 'topping-up' operation. Therefore, the priority is to provide a meal rich in energy, but easy to digest. This means that the performer should stick almost completely to carbohydrates.

A common fad with many athletes is to have honey on toasted bread with sweet tea or coffee to drink. This is quite a sound practice which it would be worthwhile for others to copy.

It must be remembered that almost anything can be eaten as a pre-event meal provided sufficient time is allowed for digestion. However, this will be discussed later.

Keeping in mind the numerous personal fads that are likely to be associated with pre-event meals, it might be wiser to suggest foods that should be avoided if eaten closer than three hours before the event. Top of this list come the grilled or fried meat dishes. These have a very slow transit time through the digestive system and are not easily converted to energy-producing substances. Also high on the priority list for avoidance are foods that are likely to produce any form of allergic response; these include shell-fish and some meat and other fish dishes. Actually, it is the protein in these foods to which the body is allergic. Salad foods such as celery are difficult to digest, mainly because of the fibrous content of the plant, and again the sportsman or woman would be wise to leave them alone until after the event. Last on my list of things to avoid is something which most people would find hard to accept. It is most unwise to take an excessive amount of the branded glucose drinks before an event. While the intention, to increase blood sugar level, is correct, they might trigger off the insulin response, which will have the opposite effect to that desired.

My final advice is to experiment, in training, with simple carbohydrate foods to establish a combination that is suitable for the individual without producing any discomfort during the event. Once the successful combination has been found it should be used for all future pre-event meals.

When to eat

The ideal time to consume any pre-event meal is between two and three hours before the competition. Protein foods will require the maximum limit, whereas the carbohydrate foods will be closer to the lower limit. Certainly, all foods should be taken well before the pre-event nerves start to show their symptoms. With very important competitions, where the mental stress is considerable, it is unlikely that the athlete will feel like eating. This is almost certainly associated with the secretion from the adrenal glands which prepares the body for the fight, but suppresses other organs and tissues of the body, including the digestive system. So in this respect nature tends to guide. On the other hand, if a meal is taken and timed just before this period of mental excitation starts, it could help to delay the 'fight' response until closer to the actual event. The controlled secretion of adrenalin is something with which the top-level performer will become familiar, and eventually master. I am certain that research into this area of body chemistry will, in the future, contribute to even higher levels of achievement.

The branded 'artificial' foods such as Nutriment, Ensure and Complan all have their place as a pre-event meal and could even be taken closer to the time of the competition than the suggested two hours. However, I do not personally recommend anything closer than the time previously stated. Nutriment tends to be rather like a flavoured milk and will certainly produce sickness if taken too close to an event where sustained movements are involved. Complan, used like a cereal or added to stock to form a soup or broth, is a good pre-event meal.

If the performer follows these simple guidelines, then there should not be any difficulty. However, I must emphasise the need to experiment during training so that this factor never presents itself as a problem on the big day.

While a lot has been written about pre-event meals, very little is documented on post-event meals. Recent research work on energy and energy replacement indicates that energy is best replenished immediately following activity and, in extreme cases, when it is delayed, the system can take up to 48 hours to be restored. Currently I am working with a top-class group of runners who I encourage to eat an apple as soon after exhaustive exercise as possible. Most people find that in the exhausted situation the appetite is not restored until several hours after the activity. However, I have found that apples and grapes are palatable very soon after activity and they do contain easily absorbed energy. While grapes probably offer the best energy replacements, they are not as convenient to transport to training sessions as an apple. It is my experience that most top-class runners will have trained probably twice within the suggested 48 hours replacement period; hence they are functioning on continually depleting energy reserves. Such a situation highlights the need for fairly frequent periods of total rest to enable the energy reserves to be replenished.

While on the subject of when to eat, the aspiring sportsperson is well advised never to eat a large meal after eight in the evening. Meals take quite a considerable time to digest and this is likely to interfere with rest and sleep.

Special diets for special events

In recent years, following a disclosure by Saltin, many marathon runners have used the carbohydrate 'bleed-out' diet prior to a marathon race. There are several versions of this diet, all of which basically involve depletion of the glycogen reserve of the body by sustained running and avoidance of carbohydrate-rich foods and fat foods, hence relying upon protein for energy; then, immediately before the event, there is an attempt to boost the reserves of glycogen by resting and ingesting 'energy-rich' foods.

The underlying principles behind carbohydrate loading are as follows.
1. During prolonged exercise, the carbohydrate reserves of the body are depleted. Energy for exercise is derived almost entirely from the

metabolism of fats and carbohydrates. Whereas the reserve supply of fats is almost inexhaustible, carbohydrates are only stored in limited amounts.

2. Once the carbohydrate supplies have been depleted, fats are used for energy. However, when fats are used for energy the efficiency of the body is reduced, which must be reflected in a reduction of training/competition times.

3. The rate at which glycogen is depleted depends upon the intensity of the work load. At very high levels of work the body obtains a greater proportion of its energy from carbohydrates.

4. The only way to obtain a complete depletion of glycogen is to exercise at an intense level so that muscle and liver glycogen stores are expended. Without depletion of glycogen, extra carbohydrates will not produce the over-compensated effect.

5. Depletion is necessary in order to stimulate fully the enzymic activity necessary for the synthesis of glycogen.

6. During the 'depletion' phase, some carbohydrates are necessary in order to facilitate the correct functioning of several important systems, for example kidneys, nervous system and red blood cell production. Likewise, during the 'loading' phase, some protein is essential for tissue repair.

7. During the loading phase, extra fluids must be consumed as a certain proportion of water is stored with each unit of glycogen. If the fluid intake is not increased other body fluids will be used, which could lead to a relative condition of dehydration.

8. For over-compensation to take place, there must be a relative period of rest during the loading phase. Hence, this must be allowed for in the eating process, otherwise it would be possible to overeat and so affect the strength/weight ratio.

9. The precise peaking effect will vary from person to person. Usually, the peak will occur between two and four days from the loading period. However, it is important to experiment before the all-important occasion, to make sure that the maximum benefit from the system has been achieved.

Many top-class marathon runners have experimented with the diet, as advocated by Saltin, and some have had considerable success. Saltin, in his original work claimed a difference of seven minutes, over a 30 km run, in favour of those who used the loading diet. Other research workers in the USA have supported these findings. The most marked effect is over the final stages of a run, when normal glycogen supplies would be very low.

The total system would appear to be as follows.

1. Seven days before the big event, the competitor takes a fast, sustained run of about 30 km to deplete the glycogen stores.

2. For the next three days he or she continues training on an almost carbohydrate-free diet.

3. For the remaining three days, including the day of the competition, he or she loads with carbohydrates.

In conversation with athletes who have used this system, the problem which emerges appears to be the 'low' feeling during the depletion phase, while training is continued. Some have suggested that it could shatter an athlete's confidence unless he or she has complete faith in the system.

More recently, some athletes have been experimenting with a modified form of the diet, using only the depletion run followed by the loading phase, without the extended depletion period. Time alone will determine the success, or otherwise, of this modification. From speaking to good physiologists, I have formed the opinion that it should be just as successful as the earlier method.

9

Ergogenic aids

Sport is now big business, with success in the chosen field bringing with it rich rewards for those fortunate enough to reach the top. With vast sums of money at stake a 'win at all costs' philosophy is often adopted. The cauldron of top-level sport encourages the participants to seek any advantage over their rivals. Initially the rivalry was man against man, competing only with his natural talents, but as time progressed the training of the endowed talents produced better results and intensified the competition. Many people now believe that top-level sport has taken over from war, with one nation striving to prove its superiority over another. Assuming this philosophy to be correct, we must remember that it has been shown in the past that in war no holds are barred. The use of poisonous gas, mass bombings, atom bombs, etc. can only be likened to the athlete who takes dope to gain an advantage. If one adds to the political considerations the total enhancement of status afforded to those successful in sport, then the scene is right for all avenues, both ethical and unethical, to be explored. This is the problem which all governing bodies of sport must now face. International sport in the twentieth century is far removed from the gentlemanly days of old, but there is one consoling thought and that is that at grass roots, sport is the same as it has always been. Completely different philosophies must be applied to those at the top and those with lower ambitions.

Every weekend thousands of people enjoy themselves playing soccer, and while the basic rules are the same, what takes place in our major grounds on a Saturday afternoon is far removed from what happens on the village green. The two are poles apart and there is no logical reason why what happens at the top level should impinge on the lower strata. I am certain that this is the basic philosophy that must be adopted by the administrators of our sport.

Ergogenic aids are basically aids which will help to produce work. They can help the speed of movement or the development of strength, delay the onset of fatigue or speed up the recovery process. If science can help to make the sick well, why should it not be used to make the fit fitter? However, with this philosophy the gulf between what is ethical and not becomes narrower as the years progress and science adds to our store of knowledge.

Even at the period of the ancient Greek Olympic Games sportsmen looked towards special foodstuffs in the hope of improving their performance. Looking through the old texts on sport we can see that the search for a 'magic' food continued and eventually led to experiments with alcohol and tobacco; are these ergogenic aids, foods, dope, drugs? And were they the forerunners of what exists today?

A fairly recent American journal lists the following preparations known to have been used by sportsmen: caffeine, camphor, cocaine, tranquillisers, nikethamide, strychnine, pentylenetetrazol, ether, digitalis, nicotinyl, alcohol tartrate, ephedrine, nicotine, nitro-glycerin, alcohol, amphetamine sulphate, epinephrine, thyocynate, ventrum alkaloids, Rauwolfia alkaloids, serpentina, potassium, citrates, bicarbonates, aspartic acid, gelatin, barbiturates, anabolic steroids – and this is by no means the complete list. It reads almost like a drug encyclopaedia. It might also suggest that the use of drugs is widespread in sport, but I am certain that this is not the case. Some drugs are undoubtedly taken at the top level merely to help tip the balance of success, but I am convinced that athletes and top sportsmen and women are not habitual drug-takers. They merely see drugs as a stepping-stone towards excellence.

It is possible to group the drugs likely to be used in sport under the following headings: tranquillisers, local anaesthetics, cardiac stimulants, cardiac depressants, anti-Parkinsonian drugs, CNS stimulants, vasodilators and synthetic hormones.

The tranquillisers, which are mainly of the Rauwolfia group, calm anxiety, relieve tension, and bring about a tranquil state of mind without impairment of the mental function. While a mild tran-quilliser might help to calm pre-match nerves, the tranquillity is unlikely to aid the fostered aggression needed for many sports, though obviously it could have a beneficial effect in such sports as pistol-shooting or archery.

Local anaesthetics paralyse the sensory nerve endings and their use in rehabilitation is certainly justified. However, their use to encourage a player to continue when injured cannot be condemned too strongly. The toxicity of the drug is not the issue at debate, but rather the extended damage likely to be caused by prolonging activity on something which has broken down.

Cardiac stimulants are a group of drugs which bring about an increase in the force of contraction of the heart and increase the blood supply to the liver, kidney and active tissues. Theoretically, they could be used to aid performance in short duration events.

Cardiac depressants are known in medical circles as Beta blockers and the layman would find it hard to believe that such drugs could have an effect upon physical performance. The use of cardiac stimulants sounds logical, but depressants quite absurd. However, performance in sport is directly proportional to the quality of work one is able to do. If, during training, a sportsman or woman is given a cardiac depressant, the level of work has to be increased. Provided the stressing agent is not too severe, adaptation will take place. When the body is released from the effect of the drug a 'super-charged' effect could result. It sounds almost like science fiction, and let us hope it remains just that.

Anti-Parkinsonian drugs are used in the treatment of Parkinson's disease where the patient finds it hard to initiate muscular movements due to loss of muscle tone. The drug improves muscle tone and aids the initiation of fast movements. To quote from Med-index: 'They [anti-Parkinsonian drugs] reduce muscular rigidity, giving improved posture, balance and motor co-ordination.'

The CNS stimulants, in the main, form the amphetamine group. Amphetamines act on the body rather like adrenalin, which prepares the body for a fight. They have a stimulatory effect upon the central nervous system, producing a state of callousness towards fatigue – a kind of Dutch courage. It has been suggested that this group of drugs has accounted for at least one death in sport.

The vasodilators improve the perfusion – or blood supply – of muscles. There are two groups, coronary and periphery vasodilators; it is probably the peripheral group which might interest sports-people. The group is derived from nicotine acid, which is known to have been detected in sportspeople.

Synthetic hormones form the last of the groups, and the one which could, and probably does, have a profound effect upon sport. These hormones fit into the complex organic compounds group known as steroids which are related to cholesterol and the lipid chain of substances. The significant preparations of this group, for sport, are the synthesised sex hormones and the adrenocortical hormones.

The sex hormones are used in sport in two different ways; one way might be considered legal and ethical, but the other is against the rules of most sports. The illegal group, known as anabolic agents, are androgenic and improve muscle and skeletal growth. If they are used in conjunction with a carefully planned diet and strength-promoting exercise, the effect upon bodyweight, strength, power, etc. is quite dramatic. But as the group is essentially the male sex hormone, its likely side-effect with women could be horrific masculinisation.

The other group is associated with the female group of hormones, oestrogen and progestogen. Most people will recognise this group as being used in the birth-control pill. Its use in sport is to adjust the menstrual cycle of women competitors so that the difficult part of the natural cycle does not coincide with top-level competition. The 'pill', taken under the supervision of a doctor, is relatively free from any harmful side-effects. It does have an effect upon the utilisation of vitamins B and C, particularly the rapid depletion of vitamin C, and this is a side-effect of which the sportswoman must be aware. It might also serve as a timely reminder that it is unwise to upset the natural balance of hormones for any reasons other than therapeutic.

More recently, it has been suggested that the pill can have a beneficial effect upon cardio-vascular response in exercise and also upon strength development. Hence, it might appear that even the pill could be termed an ergogenic aid.

The cortico-group, particularly cortisone, is frequently used in the re-habilitation of injured sportspeople, although in recent years its use has been severely criticised. If used immediately and directly on the site of a recent injury to ligament, tendon or muscle, its effect upon the healing of the injury can be most effective. However, if its use is not precise, it can have the opposite effect and can prolong rehabilitation.

If any drug or ergogenic aid has had a significant effect upon sport, that drug must surely be the anabolic steroid. It has been suggested that this drug has been used in sport since the early 'fifties. Originally, the drug was introduced to society for the treatment of anorexia (loss of appetite), post-operative treatment of patients, etc. In sport, its use is condemned; fairly substantial sums of money are being invested in testing procedures designed to detect its presence in competitors, and both men and women have been disqualified and suspended as a result of the post- and pre-competition tests. However, some see the situation rather as an attempt to close the stable door once the horse has bolted. Already, individuals or countries so motivated are researching methods to beat or cheat the tests, or to produce a more efficient product in advance of the testing efficiency. It is my belief that for a considerable period of time to come the 'criminal' will be better informed than the 'detective'.

With the situation as it is, one tragedy remains. Because the use of the anabolic steroid is illegal, it has been subject to back-street medical practice; and while its use has been known for over a quarter of a century there is little documentary evidence available on the possible long-term side-effects on sportsmen and women. There is certainly evidence of the known side-effects upon the aged and infirm, and it is certainly possible to predict likely side-effects so far not apparent. But there is very little documentary evidence to support any of these effects upon very fit, healthy men or women.

The mild incidence of jaundice, a possible diminution of libido, the odd reference to prostatism, are unlikely to deter highly motivated men. In contrast to this, there are many papers to support the positive effects upon sportsmen. To quote from one American research document, 'The data presented in the study leads to the conclusion that anabolic steroid treatment does accelerate the acquisition of muscular strength and size if accompanied by a high protein diet and severe muscular stress...significant differences, at the .01 level of confidence, existed between the anabolic and the control group in exerting muscular force.'

The first of these statements is probably the most realistic to come from any researchers in this field. Many people regard the anabolic steroid as a magic pill. This is far from the truth. Because of its effect upon protein metabolism, and a likely gluco-corticoid effect, it enables sportsmen and women to train harder and more frequently and recover more rapidly from the stress of training. But Professor Hervey of Leeds University found that anabolic steroids alone did not significantly increase the weight of rats, thus providing further evidence to show that the rumours of 'magic' properties are unfounded. It is my belief that one can only increase weight by eating more, and that one can only become stronger by the use of positive strength-promoting exercise.

The ill-informed believe that the use of anabolic steroids is restricted to those who wish to become big and perform in heavy contact sports, weight-lifting or the heavy throwing events of track and field athletics. Again, this is not the truth and I am convinced that the drugs can have a profound effect upon any power-based sport. The associated rumours of massive doses could, unfortunately, have some foundation. People tend to believe, wrongly, that more of a good thing is always better.

Blocking agents

These are substances that can mask the presence of drugs, such as the anabolic steroid group in a urine sample which is subsequently subjected to testing techniques. In 1987 the I.A.A.F. included the drug probenicid to the banned list, realising that it was being used as an agent to prevent the detection of anabolic steroids.

Blood doping

This technique came to the attention of people involved in sport following the rumours that certain very successful distance runners had used it to enhance performance levels at the 1976 Olympic

Games. The evidence is that blood is taken from an athlete, and the red cells are separated out and stored under very hygienic conditions. Then, at a later date, just prior to competition, they are returned to the donor; it would appear that there is a marked improvement in levels of performance. While it is certain that this technique is used, it is not without the risks of serious virus and organ infections associated with the risks of removal, return and storage.

As long as the rewards in sport remain high, there will always be people prepared to cheat. Perhaps a death, directly attributed to steroid therapy in sport, might bring those involved to take a more realistic view of the situation. Perhaps legalising the drug under medical supervision, since it is not addictive, monitoring and documentation might be the answer. This would certainly help medical science but not the governing bodies of sport. Anything that breaks the rules of sport must be condemned. The only true solution is a foolproof test to be administered any time or anywhere, but I sense that this is a dream of Utopia.

Away from the use of illegal drugs, there are other preparations or foods which can affect performance in sport. Alcohol, for example, can bolster courage, increase powers of endurance, suppress anxiety, aid warming-up and stimulate aggression. Alcohol therapy of this sort should not be confused with the scenes often present at the Boxing Day 'friendly' match. Caffeine is a vasoconstrictor and so increases the contractile power of the heart and stimulates the nervous system. Researchers have found that caffeine therapy can increase work output by as much as 20 per cent. It is also recognised to have an effect upon short, explosive activities, such as the throwing events in track and field athletics and certain gymnastic skills, and is certainly used in this situation.

However, I am convinced that there is a need for planned research into the legal ergogenic aids such as natural vitamins, lecethin, minerals, etc. which would help sportsmen and women avoid the hit and miss situation in which they now find themselves.

10

Training for sport

One might question the place of a chapter of this nature in a book on nutrition. The simple motor-car analogy might help to justify it. Up to this point the text has been concerned with the grade of fuel placed in the tank. However, if the engine is not tuned correctly much of the benefit will be lost. So this particular chapter is really on how to tune the engine – to make sure that both of these support systems have a chance of functioning correctly.

Training is an act of faith, which is best regarded in terms similar to a bank deposit account. The more one puts in, the more can be drawn out at a future date. If the investment (training method) is wise, the interest yields are greater.

In training, the body is conditioned to the demands likely to be made on it during competition. Hence the terms 'training' and 'conditioning' are often synonymous. To be fully prepared for one's sport five distinct areas, with a possible sixth, must be conditioned by training to produce total fitness – an ability to take on all others on a given day. Sports trainers and coaches throughout the world regard total fitness in terms of these five S factors. They are: speed, strength, stamina, suppleness and skill. Several of the factors are interdependent; for example, an improvement in strength and/or mobility could produce an improvement in speed. The factors must not be considered in isolation other than for identification.

It is simple to identify and recognise each of the factors or abilities, as they depend, to a large extent, upon natural endowment. In other words, the sportsman or woman, for his/her talents, relies as much on nature as he/she does on nurture. A well-known Yorkshire cricketer summed up the situation admirably – 'Tha can't put in what God left out'. However, though all sportspeople have a ceiling to their potential, it is the duty of every trainer, coach and sports administrator to see that, through careful nurturing, all sportsmen and women go as far as possible towards reaching their ceiling and achieving their full potential. Indeed, it is the basic philosophy of all good coaches and trainers that potential is never fully realised. This way, there is always the belief that a little bit extra will be forthcoming.

With the factors adequately recognised, what the coach or trainer really wishes to know is how to nurture the respective qualities of total performance, how each can be trained and how each responds to training. One thing is certain – there is no short-cut to success in sport; there is no magic formula, or a special type of training that could be the 'open sesame' to success. The special abilities of a sportsman or woman respond well to training and dedicated hard work, for which there is no substitute. But there must be certain conditions associated with this philosophy. The aim of training is to adapt to the stress of competition. If the stressing agent is too severe, a breakdown rather than an adaptation will take place. This is often referred to as the general adaptation syndrome. In simple terms this means that in training, one's threshold must be approached for adaptation. If training loads are kept very low or very high, adaptation to the stress is unlikely. It is the ability to manipulate both extent and intensity of training, at a particular time of the year, to bring about total adaptation, that makes a good coach or trainer.

In sport, we frequently hear that practice makes perfect. This is only true in part. Well-directed practice is a component that aids perfection. But if a performer, through lack of correct advice, continually practises the wrong movement, or the wrong training regime, then perfection will not result. This is yet another duty of the coach/trainer – to make sure that all practice sessions are constructive.

Speed

Speed, over a given distance, is determined by two factors only: leg speed and stride length. Here, of course, I am referring to the ability to run. It is this ability that is common to most of the field and court games. It is the quality that helps the athlete to be in the right place at the right time. Some sports require the performer to run at peak speed for an extended distance, while others might only call for a few speedy steps.

Leg speed
This is dependent upon the innate quality of muscle tissue and nerve impulse. A person is born with a preponderance of 'fast twitch' or 'slow twitch' muscle fibres. It is the fast fibres which are called upon to produce leg speed. Other than this inborn quality, there is the skill of the movement to be considered. The greatest inhibitor of speed is tension, so the skill to be learned is the ability to control muscular tension and relaxation. Both of these factors depend upon strength and joint mobility (suppleness). The skill factor combining the two can be taught. To help train this quality, full effort sprinting must be

performed, frequently, over a short distance. For example, a training session might be ten repetitions of a distance of 30–60 m. Less than 30 m, full-speed achievement is unlikely; more than 60 m could call upon an endurance factor. To keep the quality of speed, full recovery is essential between the repetitions. Anything that can aid the quality of the movement should be considered, such as a run down a slight incline, use of a tail-wind, use of a fast surface, being towed or paced by a machine such as a bicycle.

Stride length

Stride length is dependent upon three factors: leg length, over which the individual has no control; strength of muscles to use the levers of the leg to the full extent; and mobility of the joints of the leg to facilitate full extension.

The last two can be achieved by isolated strength and mobility exercises, which will be explained in the respective sections, such as high knee pick-up or complete ankle extension, skill drills and specific strength drills. In skill drills, the athlete concentrates upon a particular aspect of skill for a set number of repetitions. Specific strength drills include harness running (photograph 2) and hill sprints.

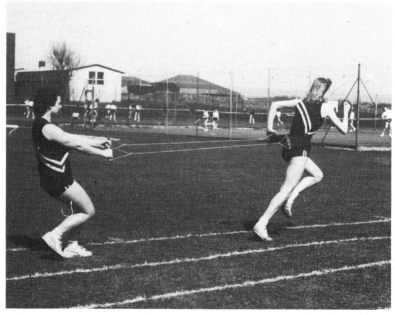

2 Harness running is an excellent way of developing specific strength

Superficially, it might seem easy to recognise speed; this is not quite true. Speed is relative – a person might look fast when placed alongside a slower person. The trainer/coach should have some method for evaluating both potential and achievement. A reliable guide is a stop-watch time for 30 m, from a standing start. A good adult man should be in the region of 3.8 sec, with about a 0.5 sec differential for a woman. Other pointers are performances in a vertical jump (jump reach test, see photograph 3), standing broad jump, standing five hops left/right. The following table illustrates approximate performance norms for good-class performers.

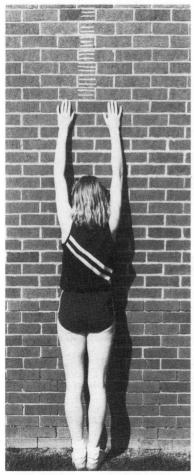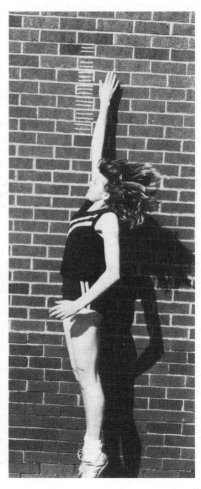

3(a) and 3(b) The jump reach test

Table 10 *Approximate performance norms for good-class performers*

event	men	women
30m	3.7–4.3 sec	4.0–4.8
vertical jump	80–100 cm	70–90 cm
broad jump	standing height + 80–100 cm	standing height + 70–90 cm
5 hops right	14.5–16.0 m	13.5 m–15.0 m
5 hops left	14.5–16.0 m	13.5 m–15.0 m

The above table also provides reliable tests for any person involved in a court or field game which calls for the ability to change speed or direction suddenly.

Strength

This is quite a confusing quality that has now forced sports trainers/coaches to recognise two quite distinct areas. They are gross strength, or the ability to exert a single, peak contraction (this is the strength characteristic of the weight-lifter); and specific strength, the ability to use a reservoir of gross strength to perform a specific jump or throw. Specific strength includes an area now recognised as 'elastic' strength and aptly termed 'plyometrics'. There is no doubt in my mind that the current high performances in certain sports, particularly track and field athletics, can be directly attributed to a better understanding of the development of this quality.

Because of its specificity, strength is most difficult to define, recognise and measure. The Olympic weight-lifter who can push 180 kg (397 lb) above his head in a single movement must surely be strong; so too, in a different sense, is the person who can propel his own body 8.90 m (29 ft 2½ in) in a single jump. Because a muscle is large, it does not necessarily mean that it is strong. The bodybuilder can have big, well-defined muscles because of an expansion of blood vessels as opposed to an expansion of muscle fibre. Strength can be measured with a dynamometer (see photographs 4a and 4b), a calibration dial in association with a spring, or a pneumatic cylinder. But these instruments are expensive to buy and vary considerably from instrument to instrument. The Olympic lifter can measure his strength against a standardised exercise, but, because of the skill factor, this is unsuitable for any other sportsperson. I believe the dictionary definition 'having powers of resistance' should convey to

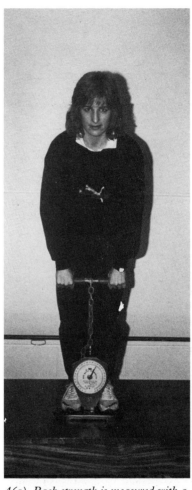

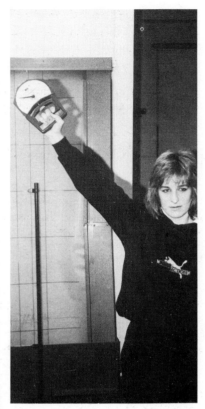

4(b) Grip strength, which reflects arm strength, is measured with a hand dynamometer

4(a) Back strength is measured with a special dynamometer. Leg strength can be measured with a similar piece of equipment

the coach/trainer and performer the correct understanding of strength. Following this, the term used for the development of strength should be 'progressive resistance training'. With this under-standing, the resistance can be the bodyweight, an elastic or spring, a weighted disc, etc. Progress can be made by increasing the resistance, as strength levels are improved.

Gross strength

The best way to improve gross strength is to exercise against a big resistance. The most convenient method for this is weighted discs (see photographs 5a–d) or use of a machine similar to the multigym (see photographs 6a–c). For maximum development one is concerned with four variables – the exercise, the grouping of exercises, the number of repetitions and the number of sets of repetitions.

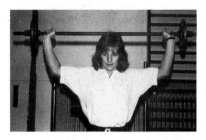 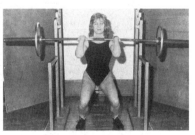

5(a) Demonstration of an arm exercise, pushing from the chest using a barbell. This exercise is performed in a seated position to isolate the legs and back

5(b) This illustrates a leg exercise – front squats using a barbell

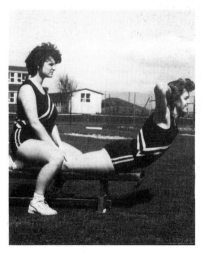 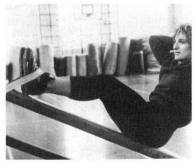

5(d) This illustrates a trunk exercise – sit-ups on an inclined bench. A weight can be held behind the head, or the incline can be increased or decreased

5(c) This shows a back curl being executed while the athlete holds her arms behind her head

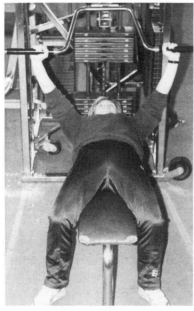

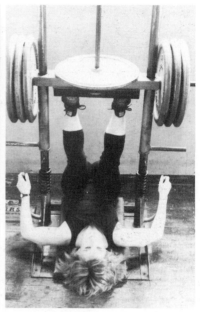

6(a) An arm exercise – the bench press – using the 'multigym'

6(b) A leg exercise using a machine. The girl high jumper uses in the region of 320kg (700lb)

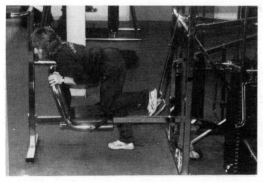

6(c) A single leg push is illustrated, using the 'multigym' leg press station

The exercise This is the basic movement such as the bench press, squat, sit-up. In the main, the exercise will bring into function a major muscle group. A number of exercises should be selected to strengthen the whole body or specific areas requiring special emphasis.

Grouping of exercises An exercise can be performed on its own as in the 'simple' system; two exercises can be linked together as in the 'combination' or 'super-set' system. The exercises are grouped together to bring about a specific strengthening effect and the system involves going direct from one exercise to another, without the customary recovery period. It is often used to promote strength endurance.

The number of repetitions A movement can be performed once, or it can be performed several hundred times. Each complete cycle of movement is termed a repetition. Generally speaking, in weight training the number of repetitions seldom exceeds twenty.

The number of sets This introduces an understanding of the 'intermittent' work theory.

A greater work-load can be achieved if short bouts of work are spaced with a period for recovery. In this particular case, an exercise might be performed for six repetitions followed by a recovery interval before the exercise is repeated, each group of repetitions being a 'set'.

By carefully manipulating these variables, relative to the season, a desired strengthening effect can be brought about. Earlier in this chapter, reference has been made to extent and intensity. Here 'extent' refers to the total volume of the combination of sets and 'reps'; 'intensity' is the value of the load, frequently measured, as a percentage of one's personal best for the exercise. Quite obviously, when the intensity of loading is high, the extent or volume of work has to be reduced.

Specific strength

Total development of gross strength will probably only assure success in the Olympic weight-lifting arena. The sportsman or woman is only concerned with usable strength, that which can be used to improve the performance of the individual. This now introduces another theory – that of transfer of training. There is only likely to be a transfer of training from one movement to another when the two movements involved call for an almost identical muscle action. The closer the similarity between movements, the greater will be the transfer of training. In this respect the sportsman or woman must consider the use of elastics, pulleys, resistance machines, etc. to aid this transfer effect (see photographs 7a and b).

To develop elastic strength, bounding activities, depth jumping, medicine ball work and similar activities must be considered (see photographs 8a and b). Again, these must be performed for a given number of sets and reps. I find the 'jumps decathlon' most helpful in promoting this quality (see Appendix B).

For the evaluation of strength, certain power weight-lifting exercises can be used. I find the power clean, the power snatch, the front squat and the bench press helpful in assessing the effect of a particular strength programme. I must emphasise that these are skilful movements and must be learned and perfected for them to be reliable, valid tests. If these tests are used in conjunction with those listed under the 'Speed' section of this chapter, then one has quite a reliable means for evaluating a training effect.

7(a)

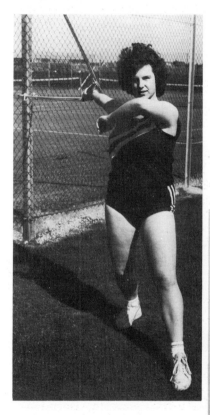

7(b)

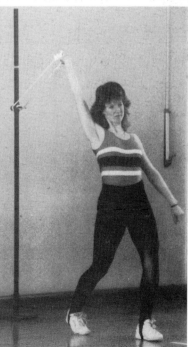

7(a) and 7(b) Elastic and pulleys can be used to aid the transfer effect between nearly identical muscle actions

8(a)

8(b)

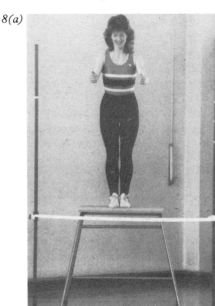

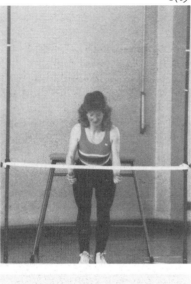

8(c)

8(d)

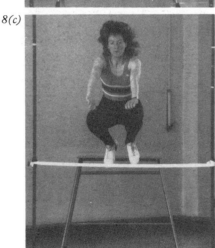

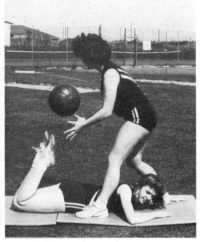

Photographs 8(a)–(c) illustrate depth jumping, a superb 'power' exercise. Here the athlete has dropped from a raised platform and has cleared a bar at 1m (3ft) from the ground. In this case, both legs have been used to provide the power. It can be done for distance and using a single leg take-off

Photograph 8(d) illustrates one of the many 'power' exercises which can be done with a medicine ball and a partner. In this situation the ball has been rolled down the back of the legs and 'flicked' back to the server by the heels

Stamina

Endurance is the term which should be used. Again, because of its specificity, this is a confusing area. In basic terms, sports coaches recognise three distinct areas of endurance: cardiovascular efficiency, local muscular endurance and anaerobic efficiency.

1. Cardiovascular efficiency This is the base, or foundation, upon which all other aspects of endurance are developed. It refers to the efficiency of the oxygen transportation system. Oxygen is required for work and is transported to the active tissues by the blood, which in turn is pumped around the body by the heart. A strong, efficient heart is a prerequisite for most sports. The efficiency of the system can be developed through sustained runs which, ideally, should be of at least twenty minutes duration. It is the sustained pressure of the work which places an overload on the heart, calling for its adaptation. Running is the simplest and the best method for developing this quality. For extra stimulation the speed can be varied, as in 'Fartlek' running, or the terrain can be varied to help relieve the boredom of exercise.

2. Local muscular endurance This refers to the ability of the individual muscle groups to perform work of a sustained nature. This is almost certainly the type of endurance required of the mountain climber or the yachtsman, where the heart rate is not necessarily raised by the level of work. This ability is best developed through circuit training employing the familiar exercises such as pull-ups, sit-ups, dips, squat jumps and burpees. Usually a circuit is performed three times, increasing the exercise 'dose' as fitness improves.

3. Anaerobic efficiency This term certainly requires a definition. Anaerobic, and its opposite aerobic, refer to the lack or presence of sufficient oxygen to perform the activity. When the level of work is low, the performer is working in the 'steady state' and there is sufficient oxygen available, through the cardio-respiratory system, to cope with the volume of work. When the level of work is high, the normal oxygen transport system cannot cope, and the performer is forced to use another energy system which involves utilising an oxygen debt capacity. This capacity varies from person to person and can be improved by training. Basically it involves the ability to cope with the high activity waste products, mainly acidic materials, which tend to have a paralysing effect upon the active tissues. Training for this quality requires the performer to do very high quality work, using an 'intermittent' approach.

A large amount of training for sport involves the use of the intermittent work principle. The early researchers in the field of work physiology found that greater workloads could be performed intermittently (a period of effort followed by a recovery period before a repeated effort) than if the work was of a sustained nature. This theory introduces four basic variables: (a) the quality of effort, (b) the duration of effort, (c) the duration of recovery, and (d) the type of recovery.

It will be seen that (a), (b) and (c) are closely linked. If the quality of effort is high, the duration of effort is forced to be short, and the recovery is likely to be long before the next period of effort.

The most common of the intermittent work systems is known as interval training. Interval training is essentially a heart conditioner, where the quality and period of effort are sufficient to elevate the pulse rate to about 180 bpm, with the recovery period sufficiently long to allow the pulse rate to drop to about 120 bpm. During the recovery interval the heart rate remains high, when there is no need for it to be so; hence an 'overload' principle is applied to the heart. The training stimulus is therefore during the interval. If the quality of effort is high, and causes the heart to beat in the region of 200 bpm, the training stimulus will occur during the period of effort, and becomes more oxygen debt work. This type of training is frequently termed tempo training.

By adjusting the four variables, specific training effects can be brought about.

Suppleness

This is an essential quality for most sports, but unfortunately it is a sadly neglected one. Children are born with tremendous mobility, but with age comes increased muscle bulk, which tends to restrict mobility. Ballet dancers always possess this quality, because from an early age they practise systematised mobility exercises which help to retain the mobility of infancy.

Mobility depends upon the dynamics of the joint, which incorporates a 'stretch reflex' mechanism that informs the mind when the extent of the movement is reached. This is partly a protective mechanism to prevent the elastic limit being breached. However, it can be over-protective, so there is a need to educate the joint continually to perform close to its optimum range of movement. Unfortunately, once the mobility of youth has been lost the joint will require a little more than gentle callisthenics even to keep the existing range of movement. To increase the range of movement, stretching exercises with the aid of a partner, or using a momentum effect, or using joint isolation, must be performed. A partner can help to move a limb gradually beyond the free limit of the movement, so educating the joint to appreciate the increased range of movement (see photograph 9a). If a weight is placed towards the extremity of the limb, and a specific exercise is performed, the momentum of the weight will take the limb beyond its free range of movement (see photograph 9b). In joint isolation work, the performer isolates the joint by placing it against a firm support such as a wall, floor, or door support, and performs a specific exercise (see photograph 9c).

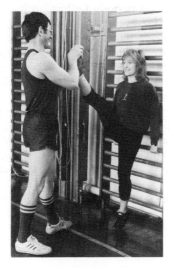

9(a) A mobility stretching movement with the aid of an 'active' partner. In this case the leg is being lifted a little higher than would normally be possible in this position

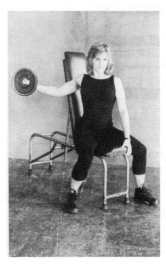

9(b) Mobility training using the 'momentum' effect of a weight and an isolated shoulder

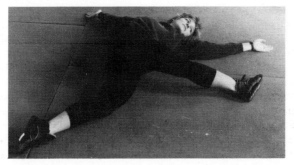

9(c) Limb isolation. The exercise performed here is to improve the mobility of the hip region

Training plans

Knowing what to do is one thing, knowing when to do it is quite a different issue. The aim of training is to produce a peak performance, or series of peak performances, at a given time of the year. It is the competitive season which dictates the phasing of training. For example, a summer sport such as track and field athletics requires a different peak period from rugby football. It is my belief, and the belief of most of those associated with training for sport, that fitness for most sports is endurance-based, and so the foundation for a training plan must be endurance-based work.

The following training plan for a track and field athlete from the northern hemisphere, wishing to peak in July/August, should help readers to understand the system for 'periodising' the year. Those who compete in winter-based sports should reverse the plan, so doing their endurance work in the summer months.

September	Period for active recovery, playing, but little systematised training.
October/November	Period where the emphasis in training is on endurance work.
December/January	Period where the emphasis in training is on gross strength.
February/March	Period where the emphasis in training is on specific strength.
April/May	Period of special event preparation.
June/August	Period of competition.

In texts of training theory, the terms microcycle, mesocycle and macrocycle will be used. These merely refer to training periods. The microcycle is a short period of time, often four days and usually less than a week. The theorists suggest that the best training pattern for adaptation to stress is:

Day 1	Easy training
Day 2	Very hard training
Day 3	Very hard training
Day 4	Rest
Day 5	As day 1, etc.

The mesocycle is a longer period of time which is composed of a number of microcycles. For example, in the training plan illustrated two mesocycles have been devoted to endurance.

The macrocycle is a still longer period of time, and is composed of a number of mesocycles. For example, the training plan devotes a macrocycle from October to January to general conditioning.

It must be emphasised that some form of evaluation should take place before, and at the end of, each mesocycle. The plan only indicates where the emphasis should be placed. Obviously speed, strength and suppleness are not completely ignored during the stamina training period.

Once a training plan has been established, it remains to prepare the detailed schedule of the microcycle – that is, what should be done on each day to provide maximum variety and, it is hoped, permit maximum adaptation.

The performer should keep an accurate training diary logging the precise training sessions, remarks on training conditions, moods, etc., and a record of all evaluation statistics together with a record of bodyweight, etc. Only by careful documentation can past mistakes be avoided. Training will always remain an empirical field because of the tremendous variation in human temperament.

It is the role of the coach to plan all training sessions in consultation with the performer, to devise the evaluation techniques and interpret the statistics, to direct and supervise most of the technical sessions, to praise when praise is due, and above all else, to console when things are not going as well as they might be. In short, the coach should be the mentor, confidant and whip![1]

To conclude I would just like to quote from Doctor Roger Bannister, the first sub-four-minute miler, in a paper published in the *British Medical Bulletin*, 1956: 'Though physiology may indicate respiratory and circulatory limits to muscular effort, psychological and other factors beyond the ken of physiology set the razor's edge of defeat or victory and determine how closely an athlete approaches the absolute limits of performance.'

---

[1] From the film 'Summer Rendezvous'

Appendix

Energy output per kilogram of bodyweight per hour for different activities from an article by Yakovlev in Track Technique *(No. 20, June 1965).*

type of activity	calories
sleep	0.93
resting, but not asleep	1.10
sitting still	1.43
free standing	1.50
class work	1.70
fast typing	2.00
slow walking	2.86
dressing/undressing	1.69
sawing wood, etc.	6.86
carrying weight of 50 kg	6.52
running 400 m/min	85.00
running 15 km/hr	11.25
boxing	7.00–13.00
skiing 15 km/hr	15.45
swimming 70 m/min	31.00
swimming 50 m/min	10.02
wrestling	12.00–16.00
rowing 80 m/min	10.00
gymnastics	4.00–8.00
horse riding gallop	7.70
cycling 20 km/hr	8.56
driving a car	1.60
hurdling	13.00–19.00
rapier fencing	9.30
sabre fencing	11.00

Index